Animal
Electroencephalography

Animal Electroencephalography

W. R. KLEMM

DEPARTMENT OF BIOLOGY
INSTITUTE OF LIFE SCIENCE
TEXAS A & M UNIVERSITY
COLLEGE STATION, TEXAS

1969

ACADEMIC PRESS   New York and London

ACADEMIC PRESS, INC.
111 Fifth Avenue, New York, New York 10003

United Kingdom Edition published by
ACADEMIC PRESS, INC. (LONDON) LTD.
Berkeley Square House, London W.1

LIBRARY OF CONGRESS CATALOG CARD NUMBER: 68-59163

PRINTED IN THE UNITED STATES OF AMERICA

Preface

Brain electric activity, recorded from the scalp or intracerebrally, is a commonly studied aspect of brain functions. Such studies have been so valuable that even wider application of electroencephalographic techniques can be expected in the future.

In this book, the term electroencephalography is used loosely to include all aspects of brain electric activity, ranging in spectrum from DC to the very rapid transients of action potentials. Although the emphasis is on potentials derived from scalp electrodes, attention is also given to potentials recorded from electrodes implanted within the brain.

Presently, investigators who study the EEG of animals fall into four main categories, and the book is intended for these people: (1) neurophysiologists, who use the EEG as a tool to assess brain function or to whom the EEG is an end in itself; (2) physiological psychologists, who usually use the EEG as an adjunct to behavioral and psychological studies; (3) biologists in a wide variety of disciplines, who use the EEG to monitor effects of the variables in which they happen to be interested; and (4) clinical veterinarians, who use the EEG for diagnostic purposes. In each category, my own research experiences impressed upon me the value of the EEG.

Ordinarily, an investigator acquires competence in this field by having personal instruction and by consulting a wide variety of books and research publications, indispensable prerequisites which require years of study. In this book I have attempted to consolidate much of the more relevant and important information, thereby reducing the time required to gain competence. It is not meant to be an exhaustive survey, but a relatively compact, single-source reference for the essentials.

Such a goal is attended by certain inevitable problems. One problem

v

is that animal electroencephalography involves many complex disciplines, and one could easily expand any chapter into an entire book. Another is that readers have diverse objectives and academic backgrounds.

The intent of the book is to provide for a diverse group of readers important general information and a rapid introduction to selected topics. With this objective, oversimplification and a degree of naivete are inevitable. The interested reader will gain sophisticated understanding only as he pursues his selected topic in depth, both by reading and by experimentation.

Some people may have become disillusioned with the utility of the EEG. This is partly because correlations of EEG with behavior are not always consistent (Chapters 6 and 7). However, any limitations on the usefulness of the EEG which may exist today are not necessarily inherent limitations of the EEG, but may result simply from our own present inability to assess its full meaning.

Electric activity is one of the most conspicuous indicators of neural function, and, therefore, study of it is logical. Electric activity can be studied at a single-cell level or on the multicellular level. The activity may be studied on either level in terms of membrane potential fluctuations or propagated action potentials (Chapter 1). Single-cell analysis has revealed the electric changes which accompany excitation and inhibition. This information, although enormously valuable, does not provide much understanding of brain function as a whole. Trying to understand brain function by study of single cells is like trying to understand a computer program by studying a transistor. Statistical laws govern brain function, and the EEG is a reflection of such processes (Chapter 1). Perhaps the best way to study the brain is by use of the double-barreled study of single cells and of the EEG. Background information for both levels of study is presented in Chapters 2–5.

The last two chapters are devoted to EEG correlates of physiologic and pathologic changes. An enormous number of the conceivable internal and external environmental conditions have been studied for their effect on the EEG, and no attempt is made to review all the pertinent literature. The objective is to summarize and discuss only some of the more important influences on the EEG. In-depth exploration of a given topic will have to be pursued by the interested reader elsewhere.

Although much emphasis is given to technical detail, this is not intended to be a technical manual. Techniques tend to change often. Moreover, the only place to really learn technique is in the laboratory. Hopefully, this book provides the necessary background to make laboratory experience more meaningful. More important than technical detail, the book strives to provide a theoretical framework which will enable the investigator to understand what he does in the laboratory.

Although the author does not assume the reader to have an understanding of modern electronics, he should have a background equivalent to that taught in a first-year collegiate physics course. An understanding of higher mathematics, although sometimes valuable, is not requisite to successful use of this work or of electroencephalographic techniques. Finally, the reader should have some experience with research and the use of precision electronic instruments.

I particularly wish to acknowledge the assistance of the experts who reviewed the chapters. Their suggestions have added immensely to the quality of the material presented. The reviewers were Dr. Rafael Flul, Department of Anatomy, University of California, Los Angeles, California (Chapter 1); Dr. D. E. Sheer, Department of Psychology, University of Houston, Houston, Texas (Chapter 2); Dr. R. H. Kay, University Laboratory of Physiology, Keble College, Oxford, England (Chapter 3); Dr. H. W. Shipton, Division of Medical Electronics, University of Iowa, Iowa City, Iowa (Chapter 4); Dr. G. Pampiglione, The Hospital for Sick Children, Great Ormond Street, London, England (Chapter 5); Dr. O. Pompeiano, Institute of Physiology, University of Pisa, Pisa, Italy (Chapter 6); and Dr. Barry Prynn, Department of Veterinary Physiology and Pharmacology, Ohio State University, Columbus, Ohio (Chapter 7). I would also like to thank Mrs. Sue Bello for her typing assistance.

College Station, Texas　　　　　　　　　　　　　　　　W. R. KLEMM
March, 1969

Contents

6. EEG CORRELATES OF PHYSIOLOGIC CHANGES

7. EEG CORRELATES OF PATHOLOGIC CHANGES

Appendix A. PROPOSAL FOR AN EEG TERMINOLOGY BY THE TERMINOLOGY COMMITTEE OF THE INTERNATIONAL FEDERATION FOR ELECTROENCEPHALOGRAPHY AND CLINICAL NEUROPHYSIOLOGY

1

Physiologic Bases of the EEG

I. Basic Elements of Nerve Cell Function

Because neurophysiology is well described in many textbooks, detailed comment is not provided here. Instead the functions relevant to the consideration of the physiologic bases of the EEG are summarized. The logical starting point in this discussion is the basic functional unit of the brain, the *neuron* (Figs. 1-1 and 1-2). Whatever the exact origin of the EEG, we must conclude that it relates in some way to the function of individual neurons.

The original studies of nerve function were conducted on the axon, the usually single process which extends from the cell body and conducts electrical impulses to the dendrites and cell body of adjacent neurons (Fig. 1-3). The early studies were devoted to characterizing the electric changes along the surface of a stimulated axon. The technique was simply a matter of placing 2 electrodes on the axon, electronically amplifying the voltage changes between electrodes, and displaying the changes on an oscilloscope. Investigators observed that biphasic voltage changes propagated along the length of the axon. The biphasic nature consisted of a propagated discrete area of negative charge, the so-called *action potential*, which as it passed the electrode proximal to the stimulation point made that electrode electrically negative to the other one. As it passed the distal electrode, that electrode then became electrically negative to the first one (Fig. 1-4). The visual display of these successive voltages was a biphasic curve.

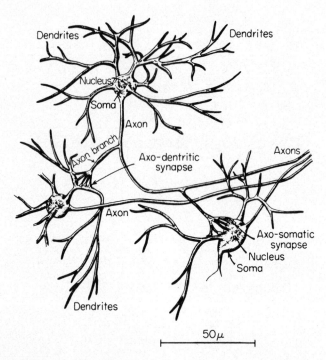

FIG. 1-1. Diagram of 3 neurons, illustrating a few of the many ways in which their processes branch and come into mutual contact. (Stevens, 1966.)

It was readily realized that electric activity was a very conspicuous aspect of axonal function, and this led to more extensive research on neuronal electric activity.

A. RESTING POTENTIALS — ACTIVE ION TRANSPORT

One of the first aspects examined was the question of charge differences between the outside and the inside of the axon. This was a crucial question, because complete understanding was not readily obtained by observing electric changes on the surface of nerves. In the earlier days there was no convenient way to insert an electrode inside an axon. The popularity of the squid axon in that era was due mainly to its large size, which permitted electrode insertion with relative ease.

Modern understanding of neuronal function derives largely from studies with sophisticated techniques involving DC amplifiers and microelectrodes. These techniques permit insertion of one electrode inside a small axon or cell body without producing any appreciable damage. Such methods reveal that the membrane of an electrically inactive neuron is *polarized*, that is, a steady potential exists across it. This DC potential ranges from about 50 to 80 mV, with the inside of the cell negative (Fig. 1–5). This membrane potential, hereafter designated as MP, amounts to a tremendous voltage, especially when considered in terms of the membrane thickness. For example, if we use a typical value for membrane thickness of 100 Å and a typical MP of 70 mV, the voltage per centimeter of membrane thickness calculates to be the astounding figure of 70,000 V. Clearly the membrane is a capacitor with great dielectric strength.

The basis for the resting MP is an asymmetric distribution of charged ions that is produced by active ionic transport mechanisms. The large amount of immovable negatively charged organic ions greatly contributes to a net negative charge inside the neuron.

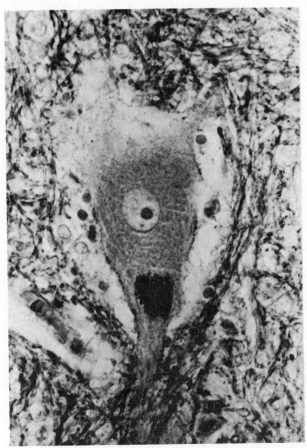

FIG. 1-2.   Photomicrograph (Nile blue stain) of a spinal motor neuron, showing nucleus, nucleolus, cell body cytoplasm, and origin of the axon containing lipofuchsin "aging" pigment. (Courtesy of Dr. Albert Few, University of Georgia.)

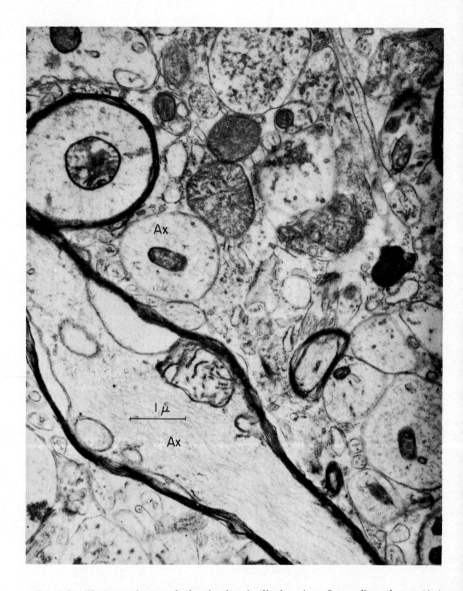

FIG. 1-3.   Electron micrograph showing longitudinal section of a myelinated axon (Ax) and cross section of several unmyelinated and myelinated axons in the medulla of a rat. Many of the axons contain mitochondria in the plane of section. Magnification × 29,500. (Courtesy of Ronald Dodson, Texas A&M University.)

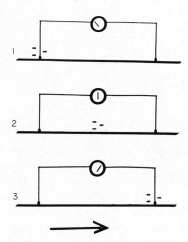

Fig. 1-4. Diagram of the passage of negative electric charge along the length of an axon in the direction of the arrow. In 1, negative charge outside the axon makes the electrode negative relative to the electrode at the right; the voltage is registered by the voltmeter between the 2 electrodes. As the outside negativity propagates, the right-hand electrode becomes negative relative to the left.

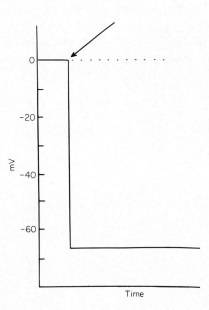

Fig. 1-5. DC potential that would be observed as an exploring microelectrode penetrated a neuron (at the time indicated by the arrow). The potential at the exploring electrode would be a steady 70 mV negative with respect to a reference electrode located extracellularly.

The origin of the charge was originally postulated by Bernstein in 1902 to result from asymmetric distribution of sodium and potassium ions. It since has been well established that in the resting state potassium is highly concentrated inside the cell and sodium is concentrated outside. Because these ions, unlike organic ions, are potentially able to move in both directions across cell membranes, they were immediately suspected of being involved in the action potential.

B. ACTION POTENTIALS

Action potentials (Fig. 1-6) are generated when neuronal membranes are sufficiently stimulated, either electrically, chemically, or mechanically. Under normal conditions, the impulses of charge are passed from the cell body down the axon, whereupon they initiate other action potentials in adjacent neurons.

The leading explanation for the ionic basis for action potentials was later found by Hodgkin, Huxley, and others, who showed that during the initial phase of an action potential the membrane suddenly becomes very permeable to sodium, resulting in a sudden influx. The sudden influx of positively charged ions reverses the polarity of the resting MP, canceling the internal negativity and actually creating a slight inside positivity. Subsequently, potassium outflux begins, and the loss of positive charge from the inside causes the inside polarity once again to become negative (Fig. 1-7). Following these ion shifts, as yet unknown mechanisms restore normal ionic balance without further significant change in the MP.

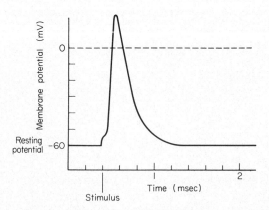

FIG. 1-6.   Illustration of a typical action potential's voltage change with time, as would be recorded from a microelectrode located inside a neuron, with a reference electrode placed outside. Stimulation of the neuronal membrane will disrupt the resting potential and cause an action potential. (Stevens, 1966.)

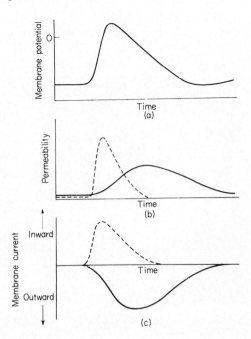

FIG. 1-7. Diagram of ionic flux changes coincident with the action potential: (a) Membrane potential fluctuations that constitute the action potential; (b) membrane permeability increase to sodium (dashed line) and potassium (solid line) that occurs during the action potential; and (c) relative amount and direction of membrane current (ionic flux) showing that due to sodium (dashed line) and to potassium during an action potential. (Stevens, 1966.)

Individual nerve cells communicate with each other via coupling of the axon of one neuron with the dendrites and cell body of another neuron. Action potentials in the afferent neuron cause changes in the resting potential in the efferent neurons. These induced MP fluctuations in the efferent neuron are called postsynaptic potentials (PSPs), discussed below.

Frequency of action potentials is assumed to be the form in which information is transmitted in the nervous system. By way of an electronic analogy, information processing in the brain can be said to be frequency modulated. The frequency of afferent impulses influences the resting potential level in an adjacent neuron, as shown in Fig. 1-8. The slow depolarizations in dendrites gradually spread to the axon hillock region which, when sufficiently depolarized, yields action potentials. On some occasions dendritic depolarizations may achieve threshold for discharging action potentials elsewhere in the neuron, but that threshold is much higher than that of the axon hillock region. Thus, the usual

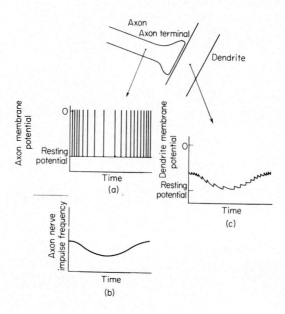

FIG. 1-8.   Translation of axonal impulse frequency into a depolarization at a dendrite: (a) Membrane and action potentials in the axon near the junction with dendrite—time scale is compressed, making action potentials appear as spikes; (b) graph of nerve impulse frequency plotted as a function of time; and (c) dendritic membrane potential changes occurring at the same time as axonal action potentials. (Stevens, 1966.)

case is for dendritic PSPs to spread through the soma to the axon hillock, where they summate to result in action potentials.

C. POSTSYNAPTIC POTENTIALS — EPSPs, IPSPs

The physicochemical processes that underlie the triggering of action potentials under normal conditions will now be considered. This triggering is initiated by impulse conduction in presynaptic junctions which in turn changes the postsynaptic membrane potential. This potential shift is due to fairly selective changes in ion permeability induced from the presynaptic terminal. When postsynaptic depolarization reaches threshold, the axon hillock membrane becomes completely unstable, resulting in a sudden sodium influx and action potentials. The depolarization is often referred to as excitatory postsynaptic potential or EPSP (Fig. 1-9). The physiology of this process has been extensively studied by Eccles and others, who also were instrumental in demonstrating that some neurons respond negatively to afferent input, that is, instead of responding with an EPSP, they actually become *hyperpolarized*, with the MP moved *away* from threshold. MPs that are hyperpolarized are referred to as inhibitory postsynaptic potentials or IPSPs (Fig. 1-10). Still another form of inhibition has been discovered, the process called *presynaptic inhibition*. This phenomenon, although not clearly understood. involves the inhibitory action of one axon terminal upon another axon terminal, perhaps by exhausting the supply or inhibiting the release of neurotransmitter chemicals.

D. CHEMICAL TRANSMITTERS — RECEPTORS

With the subject of neurotransmitters now introduced, it is appropriate to emphasize that most investigators consider the coupling between mammalian neurons to be chemical, not electrical. The evidence need not be reviewed here, but the generally accepted scheme (Figs. 1-11 and 1-12) is that impulses in a presynaptic terminal cause the release of

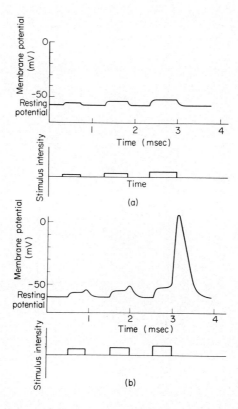

FIG. 1-9. EPSP response of a neuron to depolarizing stimuli of different strengths: (a) Small stimuli, below the threshold required for triggering of action potential, and (b) two stimuli below threshold, followed by one above threshold. (Stevens, 1966.)

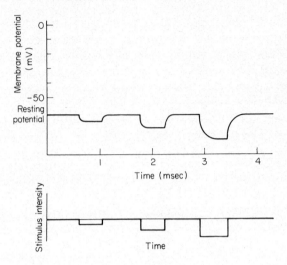

FIG. 1-10.   IPSP response of a neuron to hyperpolarizing stimuli of different magnitudes. (Stevens, 1966.)

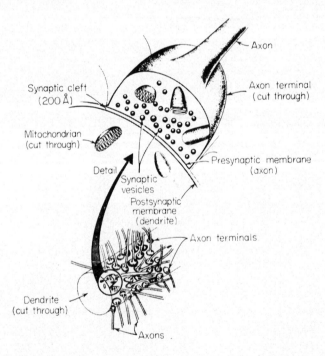

FIG. 1-11.   Diagram of the ultramicroscopic structure of the synapse wherein presynaptic vesicles release chemical transmitter that depolarizes dendritic postsynaptic membrane. (Stevens, 1966.)

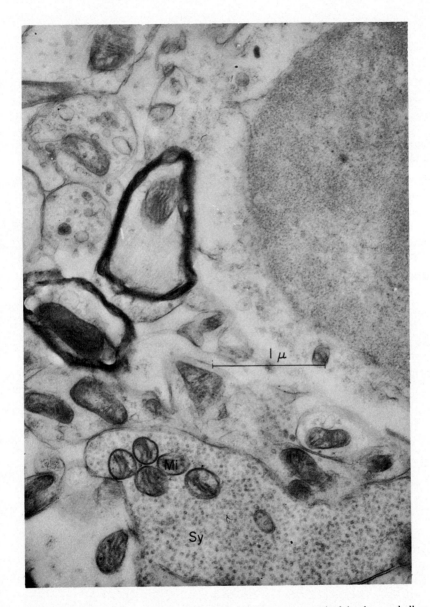

Fig. 1-12. Electron micrograph illustrating a large axon terminal in the cerebellum of a rat. Terminal contains a cluster of mitochondria (Mi) and transmitter-containing synaptic vesicles (Sy). Note patches of membrane thickening, presumed to indicate the active region of the synapse. Magnification × 31,000. (Courtesy of Ronald Dodson, Texas A&M University.)

stored transmitter substance from presynaptic vesicles. The unbound chemicals diffuse across the narrow synaptic cleft and react with compatible molecules on or in the postsynaptic membrane. These postsynaptic molecules, called *receptors,* are discrete and scattered along the membrane. Reaction of a receptor with an appropriate excitatory transmitter in some way distorts the molecular configuration within the membrane, making it selectively more permeable to certain ions and resulting in depolarization.

We have now considered the basic electric aspects of neuronal function: the ionic concentration inequality that causes resting MPs; the
on gradients, which is associated with action
f chemical transmitters which cause PSPs. It
that these elements combine in some way to
ena recorded in the EEG. The vexing prob-
ese elements is most directly responsible for
idering this problem further, perhaps we
ajor characteristics of the EEG.

II. General Nature of the EEG

A. CORTEX STRUCTURE

The brain electric activity that is recorded at the head's surface is generally assumed to originate from the cortex. The premise is that activity from deep subcortical areas is too attenuated at the surface to be recordable. One basis for this conclusion comes from such microelectrode studies as that by Brock *et al.* (1952), which demonstrated that extracellular MP fluctuations diminish greatly within a short distance from the neuron of origin. On the other hand, some EEG activity can be recorded in decorticate animals, especially over temporal and occipital regions (Cobb and Sears, 1956).

Cooper *et al.* (1965) reviewed previous studies of this question that suggested that volume conduction of subcortical potentials is insufficient for those potentials to be recordable at the surface. In their own work on humans they even showed that many transients recorded directly from the cortex did not appear in scalp recordings above the same region; generally, a transient had to be present over 2.5 cm² of cortex before it was detectable at the scalp. They also showed records where electrically evoked cortical potentials of 1–2 mV were not registered by adjacent intracortical electrodes that were only 8 mm away. Scalp attenuation of cortical voltages varied with different waveforms, ranging from 2000- to 5000-fold. In the study of dogs by Redding and Colwell (1964), simultaneous recording of scalp and intracortical potentials revealed similar waveforms in both records, but the cortical potentials were about twice the amplitude of scalp potentials.

Since the cortex is the main source of EEG waveforms, cortical structure is quite relevant to this discussion. The cortex generally contains 6 distinct layers, and although these vary somewhat in different regions, the layers are usually organized as shown in Fig. 1-13.

The previously discussed principles concerning surface attenuation of deep-seated voltages lead to the conclusion that the uppermost granular layer of cortex probably makes the greatest contribution to the surface-recorded EEG. The granular layer actually consists of densely packed dendrites that originate from more deeply situated cell bodies, the axons of which project into deeper cortical regions. The largest and

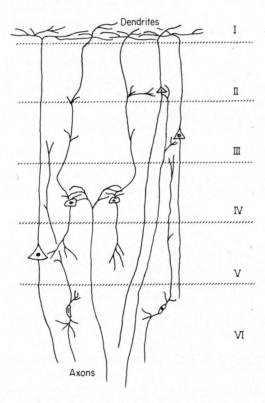

Fig. 1-13. Diagrammatic, cross-sectional representation of cell organization in the cerebral cortex. I: Molecular layer; II and III: layers of small and large pyramidal cells, respectively; IV: layer of small polymorphous cells; V: white matter and large, deep pyramidal cells; and VI: fusiform cell layer.

most prominent of these cell bodies are the so-called *pyramidal cells* in layer III, which are oriented vertically, in parallel. Many studies have demonstrated differential voltage properties in various layers of the cortex (refer to Ochs, 1965), in large measure due to the vertical orientation and to the fact that changes in a given cell's polarization do not simultaneously affect all parts of the cell equally. This principle affects the EEG waveform and is illustrated in Fig. 1-14.

The previous comments on the low level of volume conduction of intracerebral potentials should not obscure the fact that the cortex does reflect subcortical activity by means of physiologic conduction. As discussed in more detail in Chapters 6 and 7, the cortex receives afferents from many subcortical regions and is regulated in large measure by these subcortical influences. Therefore, both physiologic and pathologic

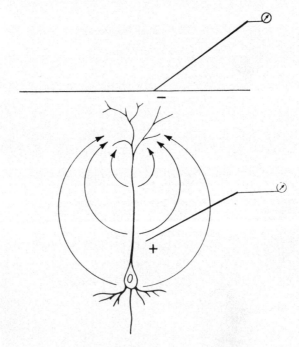

FIG. 1-14.   Diagram of the vertical orientation of cortical pyramidal cells and ionic flow in different regions. In the upper parts of the apical dendrites is a "sink," to which flows ionic current from "sources" at the axon hillock region. Current flow arrows follow engineering convention; actually, the sink is depolarized and its negative ions would tend to flow toward the axon hillock, which at this instant is polarized. The sensing electrodes near the sink (−) and source (+) would sense transient voltage differences between the upper and lower parts of the cortex. (Ochs, 1965.)

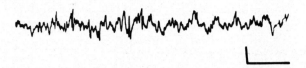

Fig. 1-15.   Sample EEG. Calibration marks: 20 μV, 1 sec.

changes in subcortical regions, by projection through synaptically related pathways, will alter cortical activity and, in turn, the activity
recorded from the scalp.

B. EEG Voltage–Time Relations

The EEG is actually a graphic plot of voltage as a function of time. The
exact nature of these waveforms is influenced by many physiologic and
pathologic conditions (Chapters 6 and 7). For introductory purposes,
however, Fig. 1-15 will serve to illustrate the more salient features of
an EEG.

Such an EEG is said to be a record of "spontaneous" brain electric
activity. Actually the term spontaneous is a misnomer and is merely
intended to denote activity present without any deliberate attempt to
stimulate the brain. Even when an investigator does not deliver sensory
stimuli, there are many influences upon cortical electrical activity:
change in membrane impedance; intra- and extracellular chemical
change; random and rhythmic synaptic transmission from cortical and
subcortical neurons; and electrotonic spread (electric field effects) from
immediately adjacent active neurons. Even neurons in surgically isolated cortex, although they exhibit long periods without activity (electric silence), often mutually interact to produce periods of activity.

As seen in Fig. 1-15, the EEG displays a variety of amplitudes and
wave durations. Although amplitudes are quite variable, it is clear that
the EEG voltages are in the microvolt range, usually about 5–75 μV in
scalp records of animals. EEG voltages are biphasic, that is, they have
both positive and negative polarities. Several factors cause this biphasic
activity: (1) volume conduction phenomena alter observed polarity; for
example, recording of a single action potential in a volume conductor
actually reveals a triphasic wave; (2) the EEG is a summation of EPSPs
and IPSPs which have opposite polarities (see Section II, C).

EEG wave durations often range from less than 1/sec to more than
100/sec, depending on the recording apparatus and physiologic conditions. There is no conspicuous periodicity; that is, waves of a given
duration do not occur with any regularity. Moreover, the record reveals

much superimposition of smaller waves upon larger, and usually slower, ones. This superimposition is actually the result of the "compounding" of different frequencies. Compounding is an inherent property of the EEG and, as pointed out in the next section, creates many problems in the analysis and interpretation of the EEG.

C. COMPOUNDING OF DIFFERENT FREQUENCIES

Compounding results because numerous cortical generators are producing different potentials at the same time. These potentials become mixed, and in the process of mixing the characteristics of the original constituents often become masked and distorted.

Some principles of compounding can be demonstrated artificially by mixing the signals from several audio oscillators and recording the combined waveforms (Walter, 1963). For example, in Fig. 1-16, 2 simple pure frequencies are mixed. When the 2 are of unequal size, only the larger is readily appreciated, serving to "mask" the smaller one. When the frequency of the larger rhythm is less than about one-fourth that of the smaller, the small waves are detected more readily as a superimposed ripple on the larger waves. In the opposite condition, when the frequency of the larger wave is about 4 times that of the smaller, the smaller waves in the compounded waveform appear to oscillate.

Waveform distortion is illustrated in Fig. 1-17, showing that when ratios of 2 rhythms are in a certain range, the rhythms distort each other. Only the frequency of the larger one is directly measurable, but some approximation can be achieved of the smaller wave frequency. Amplitude modulation can also occur. Here mixing of 3 rhythms, of which one is large and the other 2 are smaller and at equal intervals on either side of the large rhythm's frequency, causes the compounded waveform amplitude to wax and wane. Similar compounding occurs when 2 closely related frequencies are mixed together (Fig. 1-18). In naturally occurring situations, one often finds a rhythmic pattern in the EEG that increases and decreases in amplitude. One is confronted with the question of whether this is an inherent modulation of one frequency or whether several frequencies are compounded. Visual inspection, or even mathematical analysis, will not resolve the situation. However, if the wave is compounded, receiving potentials from more than one focus, the components sometimes can be separated by rearrangement of electrode positions. For example, if a pair of bipolar electrodes is arranged so that each electrode is equipotential to one focus, the potentials from that focus will be greatly attenuated (refer to differential amplifiers in Chapter 4), permitting the potentials from other foci to be more conspicuous.

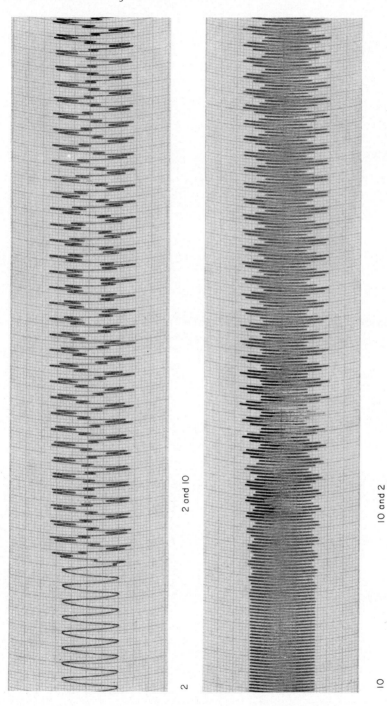

FIG. 1-16. Compounding effects of combining large and small amplitude waves of frequencies which differ about 4-fold. In top trace, addition of low-amplitude, high-frequency upon large, 2/sec waves appears as a superimposed ripple which changes its appearance with changes in phase relation to the low-frequency waves. In bottom trace, addition of low-amplitude, low-frequency waves causes an oscillating appearance of the compounded waveform.

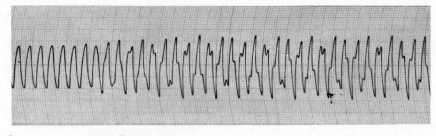

2   2 and 4

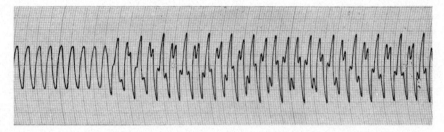

2 and 5

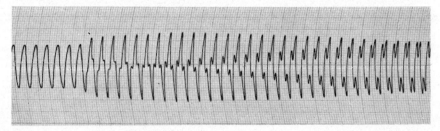

2 and 6

Fig. 1-17.   Waveform distortions produced by compounding certain ratios of rhythms. Especially if the superimposed wave is small, only the frequency of the larger one can be determined. Extent of distortion is a function of the phase relations between the 2 frequencies.

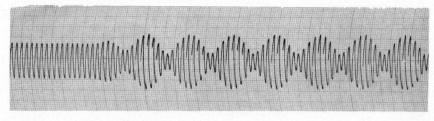

10   10 and 9

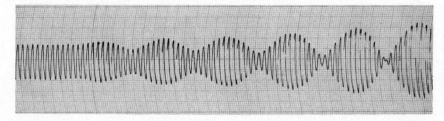

10 and 11

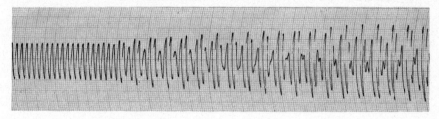

10 and 13

FIG. 1-18.   Amplitude modulation effects produced by compounding 2 closely related frequencies (top 2 traces).

III. Summation of Single-Cell Potentials

A. NEURONAL POTENTIALS

Inasmuch as the EEG is a voltage–time phenomenon, the origin of that EEG is most likely to be the voltage–time properties of single neurons: resting MPs, action potentials, and PSPs. Clearly, resting potentials cannot account for an EEG's changing voltages, although they probably are involved in the production of steady DC potentials that have been observed in the central nervous system (O'Leary and Goldring, 1964). Many years ago Libet and Gerard (1941) demonstrated a steady voltage of several millivolts when 1 electrode was placed on the surface of the cortex and another was placed below the cortex in the ventricle. Since that time many investigators have observed steady potentials (actually ultraslow potentials) in the brain, the exact polarity and magnitude depending on electrode position and physiologic state (Chapter 6). From such studies the hypothesis emerged that ultraslow potentials do indeed reflect the net state of depolarization of all the neurons involved.

To explain the voltage changes in the conventional EEG, we are left with consideration of action potentials and PSPs. It is true that central nervous system neurons do generate action potentials, often referred to as "unit potentials," of about 1 msec duration, which are superimposed on the resting MP. Eccles (1957) demonstrated that these action potentials have an ionic basis similar to that in peripheral nerve, that is, sodium influx accounts for the rising phase of the action potential and potassium outflux accounts for the falling phase.

Initially, action potentials were thought to form the basis of the EEG (Adrian and Matthews, 1934). However, most researchers now consider action potentials as an unlikely source for the EEG. The early microelectrode studies of Renshaw et al. (1940) on single cortex and hippocampal neurons gave no suggestin that the EEG was a summation of action potentials. As mentioned, action potential duration is usually about 1 msec; it is difficult to explain how these could sum to produce EEG wave durations of 10–1000 msec (100 to 1/sec). Moreover, simultaneous recording with gross electrodes and microelectrodes often show little correlation between action potentials and the slower EEG waves. However, Li and Jasper (1953) did observe some cortical neurons that stopped firing action potentials when the gross electrode EEG showed a burst of slow rhythmic waves in the same region. Also, in the study of Fromm and Bond (1967) cortical unit potentials fired fairly consistently only when the EEG ultraslow potential displayed transient shifts toward more positivity, relative to the frontal sinus reference (Fig. 1-19.). However, the published records revealed no correlation with individual EEG waves. One interesting paradox of that study was that when the ultraslow level was more negative than usual, the unit firing relation was reversed, i.e., neurons discharged only during the slow, negative transient shifts in potential (Fig. 1-20).

Even if action potentials do not account for the slow voltage changes seen in the EEG, one could still logically ask: Why do we not see action potentials in the EEG? After all, extracellular current during an action potential creates several millivolts, which should be able to be made manifest in the EEG. The answer is that action potentials *are* present in the EEG (obtained with intracerebral electrodes) but usually are not

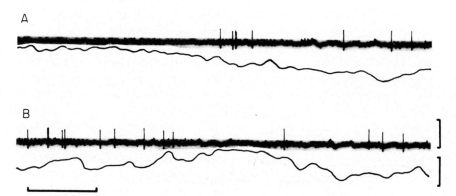

FIG. 1-19. Correlation of unit action potential discharge with ultraslow changes in potential of cortex. When the potential was between 1 and 3 mV negative (with respect to frontal reference), the neuron in the region where the EEG was recorded (lower trace of each pair) discharged only when the EEG shifted positively (negativity up). (B immediately follows A.) High-frequency components of the EEG have been electronically filtered. Calibrations: 0.5 mV for the microelectrode trace and 0.2 mV for the EEG; ½ sec. (Fromm and Bond, 1967.)

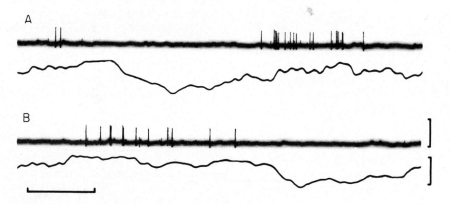

FIG. 1-20. Similar situation as depicted in Fig. 1-19, except that the resting potential was much more negative (6–12 mV negative). Under these conditions, unit discharge occurred only when EEG shifted negatively. (Fromm and Bond, 1967.)

visible because they are poorly reproduced by pen recorders and because they are masked by the slow EEG waves. However, if one were to filter out electronically the slow waves and to display potentials on an oscilloscope, numerous action potentials would be evident (Chapters 4 and 6).

Relations of the EEG to action potentials recorded simultaneously from many individual neurons have been studied by Buchwald *et al.*

(1966). The technique (Chapter 5, Section III, B, 3) involves simultaneously recording multiple unit activity and the EEG from the same electrode and permits comparing action potentials and the EEG from a given site in the brain with behavior. Such studies revealed 3 relations: (1) unit activity could change without a corresponding change in the EEG, (2) the EEG could change without an accompanying change in unit activity, and (3) only on rare occasions did both the EEG and unit activity change in correlated fashion. Such results support the conclusion that the EEG is not an "envelope" of spike discharges and that they do not *directly* correlate. More probable is the concept that the EEG represents summated postsynaptic potentials which in turn are related to action potentials in a complex, nonlinear way. We are thus led to consideration of PSPs as the source of the EEG. Actually, numerous studies have accumulated over the last 15 yr that support such a concept.[1]

The early work by Brock *et al.* (1952) pointed toward this conclusion. They reported that as microelectrodes approached a spinal motor neuron, small, fast waves were recordable. When the electrode penetrated inside a cell (as evidenced by sudden display of a resting MP), much larger fast waves appeared (Fig. 1-21). The waves had an amplitude of 0.5–1.5 mV and occurred with and without accompanying action potentials. These intracellular waves were actually spontaneous MP fluctuations that arose in the absence of intentional stimulation. Such fluctuations since have come to be inappropriately called "synaptic noise." Recent evidence suggests that the "noise" arises in part from "leakage" of transmitter but in part also from transmitter released from afferent nerve stimulation (Hubbard *et al.*, 1967).

The studies by Li and Jasper (1953) involved microelectrode recordings of brain neurons, but the experiments did not employ DC amplifiers, making it impossible to ascertain whether recorded potentials came from extracellular fluids or from inside neurons. Nonetheless, important observations were made. For example, single neurons in the cortex displayed a slow and rhythmic activity, similar to that simultaneously recorded from gross electrodes at the surface (Fig. 1-22). They also observed slow waves of about 1 mV amplitude that were mixed with action potentials when recorded by the same electrode. The

---

[1]Brock *et al.* (1952); Jung *et al.* (1952); Li *et al.* (1952); Albe-Fessard and Buser (1953); Li and Jasper (1953); Verzeano and Calma (1954); Li (1956a,b, 1961, 1963); Phillips (1956, 1961); Verzeano and Negishi (1960); Purpura and Housepian (1961); Purpura *et al.* (1961, 1964); Elul (1962, 1966); Klee and Lux (1962); Li and Chou (1962); Lux and Klee (1962); Creutzfeldt and Meisch (1963); Creutzfeldt *et al.* (1966a,b); Lux and Nacimiento (1963); Sawa *et al.* (1963); Stefanis (1963); Fujita and Sato (1964); Purpura and Shofer (1964); Jasper and Stefanis (1965).

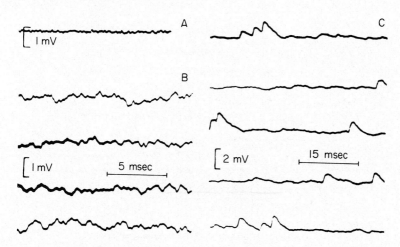

F ɪɢ. 1-21.   Illustration of MP fluctuations recorded with microelectrodes implanted in and near spinal motor neurons in cats. A: Electrode extracellular, but far from neuron; B: a series of traces taken when electrode was still extracellular but near neuron; and C: a series of intracellular MP fluctuations. (Brock *et al.*, 1952.)

only clear relationship between the two was that action potentials, when present, occurred only on the depolarizing phase of the slow waves. Another important observation was that the slow waves persisted, even after action potentials were abolished by asphyxia or anesthesia. From their results, Li and Jasper postulated that these single unit slow waves were synaptic MPs and that these contributed to the grossly recorded EEG.

The implications of Li and Jasper's study were confirmed in subsequent intracellular microelectrode studies. Phillips (1956), for example, studied intracellular activity in single cerebral cortex cells and observed MP fluctuations. He reported that MP fluctuations occasionally were accompanied by action potentials originating on the depolarizing phase of the MP.

Fujita and Sato (1964) correlated intracellular hippocampal activity with simultaneously grossly recorded hippocampal EEG (Fig. 1-23). They found that the MP fluctuated in synchrony with the EEG. Their unit records revealed slow waves with amplitudes of about 25 mV, which was about 100 times greater than that noted in records obtained from gross recording.

Another unique EEG pattern, so-called "spindles" from pyramidal tract neurons, has been found to correlate with the 4–17 mV intracellular MP fluctuations (Jasper and Stefanis, 1965). The correlation was independent of whether a discharge of action potentials occurred on the

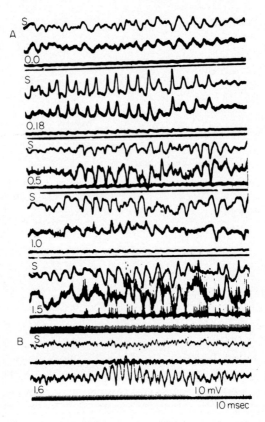

Fig. 1-22.   Simultaneously recorded slow waves from the cortex surface (S) and from microelectrodes implanted at various depths. The first line of each record was taken with a large electrode on the pial surface; the second and third lines were taken with microelectrodes through different time-constant amplifiers. A is from one cat and B is from another. (Li and Jasper, 1953.)

depolarization phase of the MP. Results also indicated that intracellular MP fluctuations were both excitatory and inhibitory.

More recently, similar results have been reported by Elul (1964, 1969). He recorded intracellular slow waves of 5–15 mV, the frequencies of which corresponded well with those in EEG records taken from the same region, both during sleep and arousal states.

All of the foregoing evidence supports the hypothesis that the EEG is a summation of the voltages produced by the MP fluctuations of individual neurons. The amplitude discrepancy (EEG waves are about 10–150 μV) can be explained by the Ohm's law relation between voltage and resistance. Because transmembrane resistance is high, voltages developed by currents through the membrane would be high. Conversely, since resistances in extracellular fluids are relatively low, voltages developed by currents through it would be low. EEGs recorded from gross extracellular electrodes register the voltages developed by currents flowing through extracellular fluids. Elul (1969) concludes that the evidence suggests that extracellular fluids have a resistance of about one one-hundredth that of nerve membranes and that this is consistent with the idea that EEG voltages come from MP oscillations of individual neurons.

Evidence also has been provided (Elul, 1962) to show that single neurons do produce extracellular currents that are sufficient to permit registration of EEG voltages. With a pair of extracellular microelectrodes, 30 μ apart, Elul recorded spontaneous activity that looked like an EEG (Fig. 1-24). He also demonstrated that activity at one electrode was not necessarily present at the other. This suggests that the potential fields of a single neuron do not extend much beyond a radius of 30 μ.

One apparent difficulty with the MP-fluctuation theory is that several investigators have noted MP changes that were out of phase with the simultaneously recorded surface waves. Creutzfeldt *et al.* (1966a,b) have

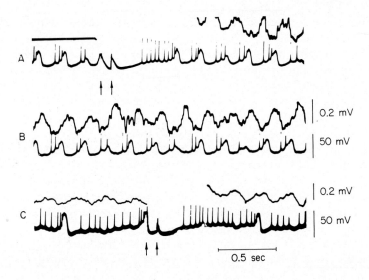

FIG. 1-23.   Illustration of intracellular MP fluctuations that correspond to grossly recorded "theta rhythm" of hippocampus. EEGs (upper traces) were taken from pyramidal cell layer, and intracellular records (lower traces) were taken from within individual cells in that layer. A and B were taken from the same cell and C from another. Upward arrows indicate time of stimulation of collaterals that produced transient hyperpolarization. (Fujita and Sato, 1964.)

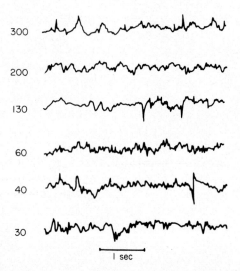

Fig. 1-24. EEG-like activity recorded from 2 bipolar electrodes implanted 600–900 μ in the cerebral cortex. Numbers on the left indicate interelectrode distance in microns. (Elul, 1962.)

helped to resolve this dilemma. They cite numerous studies that reported apparently conflicting data, some suggesting EPSP associated with surface positive waves and others suggesting IPSP association. Other workers have reported either EPSPs or IPSPs in association with surface negative waves. The explanation for these variable results is based on recalling that cortical cells are vertically oriented in the cortex, with apical dendrites projecting to the surface. This orientation, combined with variable origins of MP changes on the cell and current flow rate and direction, provide several mechanisms that influence the type of potential that a surface electrode "sees." For example, if the soma is rapidly depolarized, the surface will be initially positive, subsequently followed by surface negativity as current flow progresses. On the other hand, a fast hyperpolarization of the soma will cause an initial surface negativity before the charge affects the whole cell.

We come now to the question: Are these MP fluctuations the same as PSPs that have been so well studied in neurons located outside the brain? Such a conclusion seems reasonable, although brain neurons have not been as amenable to the thorough study that has been performed on neurons located outside the brain. Brain neuron PSPs, of both excitatory and inhibitory types, have been observed. The magnitude of the MP changes is similar to that noted in other neurons. Action potentials are usually generated on the depolarizing phase of EPSPs. As in neurons outside the brain, not all EPSPs result in action potentials.

The inconsistent relation between EPSP magnitude and discharge of action potentials suggests that intracellular waves are not linearly related to action potentials (Adey, 1966). Perhaps the threshold for action potentials is not solely dependent upon the magnitude of depolarization but also on other, as yet unknown, properties of the cell.

The failure of some, even large, EPSPs to trigger action potential discharge indicates that EEG voltages occur that do not represent "information" in the sense of conducted impulses. However, all the PSPs represent information in the sense that they are temporally and spatially summing input from other neurons. This information is no doubt mediated by quantal release of neurotransmitters; it is possible that some of the chemical release results from "leakage" from presynaptic vesicles when action potentials are not being generated in the presynaptic neurons.

Because brain neurons exhibit EPSPs and IPSPs, we can readily appreciate the importance of synaptic interactions. If the number of afferent impulses to a brain neuron fluctuates, similar fluctuation could be expected to develop in neurotransmitter release by that neuron. Consequently, there would be fluctuations in the MP of adjacent neurons that respond to that transmitter. Similar processes occurring in all cortical cells would combine to form what we call the EEG.

Such reasoning permits some speculative correlation of the time course of MP changes with that of EEG waves. If many neurons were being activated by transmitter in a random time pattern, the sum of these MPs would result in an EEG that has many short-duration, low-voltage waves; this pattern is referred to as desynchronized, and it is usually associated with alert behavior (Chapter 6). Conversely, if many neurons were activated in unison, the sum of their MPs would create an EEG with few long-duration, high-voltage waves; this pattern is called synchronized, and it is usually associated with sedated behavior. Elul (1969) reports that the time course of PSPs in a *single cell* correlates well with EEG desynchrony and synchrony. During a synchronous EEG, for example, PSPs in the cortical cell had long time courses, indicative of synchronous release of transmitter in the presynaptic terminals impinging on that cell.

The postulate that transmitter release rate and timing is correlated with the EEG is also supported by observations that EEG desynchrony is associated with an increased release of acetylcholine in the neocortex (reviewed by Jasper, 1966). This presumably results from the discharge of more action potentials. If the discharges are relatively unsynchronized, there would be less temporal and spatial summation, resulting in a faster decay of postsynaptic potentials, which is equivalent to faster frequency MP fluctuations. On the other hand, atropine blocks acetylcholine effects on cortical neurons and at the same time produces a synchronized EEG. Perhaps the EEG effect results from more synchronized discharges (not necessarily fewer) and more summation of synaptic potentials, leading to higher voltage, longer duration MP fluctuations.

Membrane potential fluctuations in brain tissue may have a mechanism similar to the so-called miniature end-plate potentials (MEPPs) of myoneural junctions. These MEPPs have been widely studied (reviewed by Ochs, 1965). Intracellular microelectrodes placed inside a muscle fiber near the end-plate region exhibit small (about 5–35 mV) transient depolarizing potential changes. Although the amplitude is about the same as that of cortical neurons, the frequency is much faster, each MEPP having a duration of 3–4 msec. Each MEPP appears to result from a quantal release of acetylcholine from the axon terminals; successive MEPPs summate to form the end-plate potential (EPP) which, if a critical level of depolarization is reached, is the prelude to the action potential of a muscle fiber. Membrane potential fluctuations similar to the MEPPs of skeletal muscle also have been observed in smooth muscle. They differ primarily in that the smooth muscle potentials occur more slowly, on the order of once or twice a second.

As pointed out by Adey (1966), there are still many questions to be resolved in connection with this theory on the origin of the EEG. For example, many areas of the brain exhibit regional differences in MP fluctuations and in their EEG; the EEG from human occipital cortex often contains rhythmic 8–12/sec activity (see also Chapter 3, Section VI, C); the hippocampus often exhibits 4–7/sec activity; and the amygdala often discharges 40/sec activity. Other questions involve the ways in which various EEG generators are coupled with each other and how they mutually interact.

B. GLIAL POTENTIALS

The glial cells, astrocytes, oligodendrocytes, and microglia, serve as the connective tissue of the central nervous system. They are at least as numerous as neurons and, depending on how counting is done, are often much more numerous. Unfortunately, the physiology of glial cells is poorly understood, although the concept is emerging that they influence the transfer of chemicals and energy across neuronal membranes (Hydén, 1960; Svaetichin et al., 1961; Wendell-Smith et al., 1965; Hertz, 1965).

Although usually overlooked as contributors of potential to the EEG, glial cells do exhibit electric properties that may be relevant to the origin of the EEG.

Recent microelectrode studies in amphibians indicate that glial cells have large resting potentials but that they do not yield action potentials when the membrane is depolarized. Significantly, glial cells have been shown to exhibit very slow, graded depolarizations (up to a maximum of 48 mV) during discharge of adjacent neurons (Figs. 1-25 and 1-26). The depolarization begins about the time that neuronal discharge is ending. Clearly, the magnitude of such MP fluctuations in glia is sufficient to be manifest in the EEG. The decay of glial potentials, however, is much slower than that of neuronal action potentials, with a half-time of about

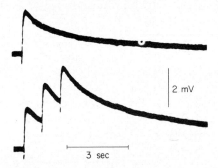

FIG. 1-25.   Glial cell depolarization produced by nerve impulses in the *Necturus* optic nerve. MP recorded with an intracellular electrode. Upper trace: depolarization following a nerve volley rises to a peak in about 150 msec and declines with a half-time of about 2 sec. Lower record: 3 stimuli at 1-sec intervals, showing summation of glial depolarization. (Orkand *et al.*, 1966.)

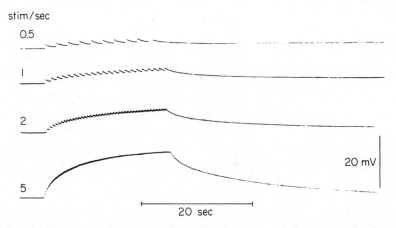

FIG. 1-26.   Summation of glial depolarization as a function of frequency of stimulation of adjacent neuron. Four trains of electric stimuli at 0.5, 1, 2, and 5/sec for about 20 sec applied to the eye end of a *Necturus* optic nerve. (Orkand *et al.*, 1966.)

2 sec. Because electric stimulation of glial cells does not initiate MP changes, it is suspected that in natural conditions glial depolarization is triggered by a chemical agent, possibly potassium, released from discharging neurons. Evidence for the potassium theory includes observations that changing extracellular potassium concentrations changes the glial MP (Kuffer et al., 1966; Orkand et al., 1966).

Elul (1969) has obtained intracellular potentials from glial cells and observed no MP fluctuations or action potentials as are found in neurons. These observations would seem to rule out any glial contribution to the conventional frequency band of the EEG of about 1–60 cps. However, glia most likely do contribute to slower potentials outside the conventional EEG frequency band.

IV. Conclusions

The evidence presented concerning the genesis of the EEG, although still far from complete, is sufficient to conclude that the EEG is a very sensitive indicator of the most fundamental functions of brain tissue. Although derived primarily from the cortex, the EEG is an indirect monitor of many subcortical brain areas that regulate cortical activity. The EEG is a random sum of membrane potential fluctuations, which in the case of neurons are known to result from transmitter–receptor interactions, which in turn result from action potential discharge. Thus, the whole gamut of information-processing mechanisms of the brain is represented in the complex voltage–time relations in the EEG.

The EEG is a summed composite of all the EPSPs and IPSPs within the pickup range of the electrodes. The EEG does not directly reveal the extent of active inhibition (IPSPs). For example, a desynchronized EEG could result simply from EPSPs or from decreased IPSP activity (disinhibition) or both. A synchronous EEG obviously would indicate a decrease in EPSP activity (disfacilitation) and probably would suggest an increase in IPSP activity (active inhibition), which would serve to pace certain circuits synchronously. These speculations are indicative of the present stage of our understanding in which we must synthesize concepts derived from results of single-cell studies. This subject is being investigated today in many laboratories.

Any utilitarian limitations of the EEG that exist are a reflection not on an inherent lack of meaningfulness of the EEG but on our own inabilities to extract the meaning. Thus, the EEG, rather than ultimately being relegated to the role of a scientific novelty, should become even more crucial in future brain research as we become better able to discern the full spectrum of its significance.

REFERENCES

Adey, W. R. (1966). Neurophysiological correlates of information transaction and storage in brain tissue. *In* "Progress in Physiological Psychology" (E. Stellar and J. M. Sprague, eds.), Vol. 1, pp. 1–43. Academic Press, New York.

Adrian, E. D., and Matthews, B. H. C. (1934). The interpretation of potential waves in the cortex. *J. Physiol. (London).* **81**, 440–471.

Albe-Fessard, D., and Buser, P. (1953). Exploration de certaines activités du cortex moteur du chat par microélectrodes; derivations endosomatiques. *J. Physiol. (Paris)* **45**, 14–16.

Brock, L. G., Coombs, J. S., and Eccles, J. C. (1952). The recording of potentials from motorneurons with an intracellular electrode. *J. Physiol. (London)* **117**, 431–460.

Buchwald, J. S., Halas, E. S., and Schramm, S. (1966). Relationships of neuronal spike populations and EEG activity in chronic cats. *Electroencephalog. Clin. Neurophysiol.* **21**, 227–238.

Cobb, W., and Sears, T. A. (1956). The superficial spread of cerebral potential fields. Some evidence provided by hemispherectomy. *Electroencephalog. Clin. Neurophysiol.* **8**, 717–718.

Cooper, R., Winter, A. L., Crow, H. J., and Walter, W. G. (1965). Comparison of subcortical, cortical and scalp activity using chronically indwelling electrodes in man. *Electroencephalog. Clin. Neurophysiol.* **18**, 217–228.

Creutzfeldt, O. D., and Meisch, J. J. (1963). Changes of cortical neuronal activity and EEG during hypoglycemia. *Electroencephalog. Clin. Neurophysiol.* Suppl. 24, 158–170.

Creutzfeldt, O. D., Watanabe, S., and Lux, H. D. (1966a). Relations between EEG phenomena and potentials of single cortical cells. I. Evoked responses after thalamic and epicortical stimulation. *Electroencephalog. Clin. Neurophysiol.* **20**, 1–18.

Creutzfeldt, O. D., Watanabe, S., and Lux, H. D. (1966b). Relations between EEG phenomena and potentials of single cortical cells. II. Spontaneous and convulsoid activity. *Electroencephalog. Clin. Neurophysiol.* **20**, 19–37.

Eccles, J. C. (1957). "The Physiology of Nerve Cells." Johns Hopkins Press, Baltimore, Maryland.

Elul, R. (1962). Dipoles of spontaneous activity in the cerebral cortex. *Exptl. Neurol.* **6**, 285–299.

Elul, R. (1964). Specific site of generation of brain waves. *Physiologist* **7**, 125.

Elul, R. (1969). Brain waves: Intracellular recording and statistical analysis help clarify their physiological significance. *In* "Data Acquisition in Medical Biology" (K. Enslein, ed.), Vol. 5. Pergamon Press, Oxford (in press).

Fromm, G. H., and Bond, H. W. (1967). The relationship between neuron activity and cortical steady potentials. *Electroencephalog. Clin. Neurophysiol.* **22**, 159–166.

Fujita, Y., and Sato, T. (1964). Intracellular records from hippocampal pyramidal cells in rabbit during theta rhythm activity. *J. Neurophysiol.* **27**, 1011–1025.

Hertz, L. (1965). Possible role of neuroglia: A potassium-mediated neuronal–neuroglial–neuronal impulse transmission system. *Nature* **206**, 1091–1094.

Hubbard, J. I., Stenhouse, D., and Eccles, R. M. (1967). Origin of synaptic noise. *Science* **157**, 330–331.

Hydén, H. (1960). The neuron. *In* "The Cell" (J. Brachet and A. E. Mirsky, eds.), Vol. 4, pp. 215–324. Academic Press, New York.

Jasper, H. H. (1966). Pathophysiological studies of brain mechanisms in different states of consciousness, *In* "Brain and Conscious Experience" (J. C. Eccles, ed.), pp. 256–282. Springer, Berlin.

Jasper, H. H., and Stefanis, C. (1965). Intracellular oscillatory rhythms in pyramidal tract neurons in the cat. *Electroencephalog. Clin. Neurophysiol.* **18**, 541–553.

Jung, R., von Baumgarten, R., and Baumgartner, G. (1952). Mikroableitungen von einzelnen Nervenzellen im optischen Cortex der Katze: Die lichtaktivierten B-Neurone. *Arch. Psychiat. Nervenkrankh.* **189**, 521–539.

Klee, M. R., and Lux, H. D. (1962). Intracelluläre Untersuchungen über den Einfluss hemmender Potentiale im motorischen Cortex. II. Die Wirkungen elektrischer Reizung des Nucleus caudatus. *Arch. Psychiat. Nervenkrankh.* **203**, 667–689.

Kuffer, S. W., Nicholls, J. G., and Orkand, R. K. (1966). Physiological properties of glial cells in the central nervous system of amphibia. *J. Neurophysiol.* **29**, 768–787.

Li, C.-L. (1956a). Facilitatory effect of stimulation of unspecific thalamic nucleus on cortical sensory neuronal responses. *J. Physiol. (London)* **131**, 115–124.

Li, C.-L. (1956b). The inhibitory effect of stimulation of the thalamic nucleus on neuronal activity in the motor cortex. *J. Physiol. (London)* **133**, 40–53.

Li, C.-L. (1961). Cortical intracellular synaptic potentials. *J. Cellular Comp. Physiol.* **58**, 153–167.

Li, C.-L. (1963). Cortical intracellular synaptic potentials in response to thalamic stimulation. *J. Cellular Comp. Physiol.* **61**, 165–179.

Li, C.-L., and Chou, S. N. (1962). Cortical intracellular synaptic potentials and direct cortical stimulation. *J. Cellular Comp. Physiol.* **60**, 1–16.

Li, C.-L., and Jasper, H. H. (1953). Microelectrode studies of the electrical activity of the cerebral cortex in the cat. *J. Physiol. (London)* **121**, 117–140.

Li, C.-L., McLennan, H., and Jasper, H. H. (1952). Brain waves and unit discharges in cerebral cortex. *Science* **116**, 656–657.

Libet, B., and Gerard, R. W. (1941). Steady potential fields and neurone activity. *J. Neurophysiol.* **4**, 438–455.

Lux, H. D., and Klee, M. R. (1962). Intracelluläre Untersuchungen uber den Einfluss hemmender Potentiale im motorischen Cortex. I. Die Wirkung elektrischer Reizung unspezifischer Thalamuskerne. *Arch. Psychiat. Nervenkrankh.* **203**, 648–666.

Lux, H. D. and Nacimiento, A. C. (1963). Membranpotentialänderungen von Zellen des motorischen Cortex nach Reizung im spezifischen Thalamus. *Arch. Ges. Physiol.* **278**, 66.

Ochs, S. (1965). "Elements of Neurophysiology." Wiley, New York.

O'Leary, J. L., and Goldring, S. (1964). D-C potentials of the brain. *Physiol. Rev.* **44**, 91–125.

Orkand, R. K., Nicholls, J. G., and Kuffer, S. W. (1966). Effect of nerve impulses on the membrane potential of glial cells in the central nervous system of amphibia. *J. Neurophysiol.* **29**, 788–806.

Phillips, C. G. (1956). Intracellular records from Betz cells in the cat. *Quart. J. Exptl. Physiol.* **41**, 58–69.

Phillips, C. G. (1961). Some properties of pyramidal neurones of the motor cortex. Ciba Found. Symp. *The Nature of Sleep.* pp. 4–29.

Purpura, D. P., and Housepian, E. M. (1961). Alteration in corticospinal neuron activity associated with thalamocortical recruiting responses. *Electroencephalog. Clin. Neurophysiol.* **13**, 365–381.

Purpura, D. P., and Shofer, R. J. (1964). Cortical intracellular potentials during augmenting and recruiting responses. I. Effects of injected hyperpolarizing currents on evoked membrane potential changes. *J. Neurophysiol.* **27**, 117–132.

Purpura, D. P., Cohen, B., and Marini, G. (1961). Generalized neocortical responses and corticospinal neuron activity. *Science* **134**, 729–730.

Purpura, D. P., Shofer, R. J., and Musgrave, F. S. (1964). Cortical intracellular potentials during augemting and recruiting responses. II. Patterns of synaptic activities in pyramidal and nonpyramidal tract neurons. *J. Neurophysiol.* **27**, 133‑151.

Redding, R. W., and Colwell, R. K. (1964). Verification of the significance of the canine electroencephalogram by comparison with the electrocorticogram. *Am. J. Vet. Res.* **25**, 857‑861.

Renshaw, B., Forbes, A., and Morrison, B. R. (1940). Activity of isocortex and hippocampus: Electrical studies with microelectrodes. *J. Neurophysiol.* **3**, 74‑105.

Sawa, M., Maruyama, N., and Kaji, S. (1963). Intracellular potential during electrically induced seizures. *Electroencephalog. Clin. Neurophysiol.* **15**, 209‑220.

Stefanis, C. N. (1963). Relations of the spindle waves and the evoked cortical waves to the intracellular potentials in pyramidal motor neurons. *Electroencephalog. Clin. Neurophysiol.* **15**, 1054.

Stevens, C. E. (1966). "Neurophysiology: A Primer." Wiley, New York.

Svaetichin, G., Laufer, M., Mitarai, G. Fatehchand, R., Vallecale, E., and Viggega, J. (1961). Glial control of neuronal networks and receptors. *In* "The Visual System: Neurophysiology and Psychophysics," pp. 445‑456. Springer, Berlin.

Verzeano, M., and Calma, I. (1954). Unit activity in spindle bursts. *J. Neurophysiol.* **17**, 417‑428.

Verzeano, M., and Negishi, K. (1960). Neuronal activity in cortical and thalamic networks. *J. Gen. Physiol.* **43**, 177‑195.

Walter, W. G. (1963). Technique-interpretation. *In* "Electroencephalography" (J. D. N. Hill and G. Parr, eds.), pp. 65‑98. Macmillan, New York.

Wendell-Smith, C. P., Blunt, M. J., Baldwin, F., and Paisley, P. B. (1965). Neurone-satellite cell relationship. *Nature* **205**, 781‑782.

2

Electrodes, Characteristics and Usage

I. Electrode Characteristics

A. Physical Chemistry of Electrodes

Electrodes generally transduce the ionic flow in tissue to electron flow in wiring that supplies the input of amplifiers. This conversion of ionic flow into an analagous electron flow is a complicated process, and the character of this electrochemical system has important influences upon the quality of transduction.

The electrode–tissue interface forms an electric battery in that potential is created between tissue and electrode. The relative rating in this respect of various metals can be found in tables of electrode potentials in a physics text. These potentials are essentially of the DC type. In bioelectric recording, if 2 electrodes create the same electrode potential with tissue, there is no difference between them. Because biologic amplifiers amplify only *difference* of potential, such electrode potentials would not be recorded. As a practical matter, however, it is very difficult to match electrodes so that they create exactly the same electrode potential. Many of these electrode potentials are on the order of 1 V or more, and it is obviously difficult to match 2 such electrodes so that their voltages cancel each other within microvolts. The common solution is to put capacitors in the amplifier input to block all DC current. Although this prohibits recording of biologic DC potentials, it minimizes electrode potentials and is an acceptable practice in the recording of the conventional EEG. If DC potentials need to be recorded, the electrodes must be matched carefully and any remaining potential canceled by amplifier balance controls.

Chemically, the electrode-potential phenomenon is well understood; the type of metal electrode and the type and concentration of ions in the

34

fluid medium determine the magnitude of the potential. The potential originates because electrode atoms dissociate, forming positive ions and free electrons; the charge separation creates a battery. The stability of an electrode potential is logarithmically dependent upon the concentration of electrode material in the area adjacent to the electrode, as quantified by the Nernst equation. This ionic concentration is influenced by many variables in tissue and, consequently, potentials fluctuate, producing severe artifacts in the recordings (Fig. 2-1).

Silver electrodes, for example, dissociate in tissue to form positive silver ions and free electrons. The positive ions react with tissue negative ions, such as chloride, to form an irregular film of silver chloride on the electrode. Thus, there are complex reactions occurring that achieve equilibrium and steady electrode potentials with great difficulty because the equilibrium is subject to so many variables. Clearly, any change in ions in the electrode vicinity will disrupt equilibrium and the steady potential, causing electric noise in the recording. The most serious disruption of equilibrium is caused by physical motion of fluids around the electrode, stirring the solution of silver ions, and changing their

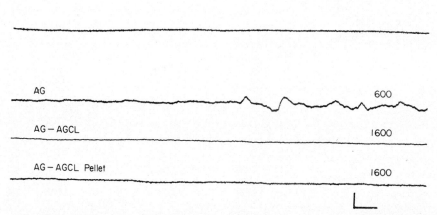

FIG. 2-1. Comparison of electrode noise with electrode pairs imbedded in electrode jelly. Top half of figure illustrates instrument noise with each amplifier recording from the same shorted input. Bottom half illustrates recordings taken from silver EEG electrodes (Grass Instrument Company) and from silver–silver chloride pellets (Beckman Instrument Company). Interelectrode resistances in DC ohms are shown for each pair; the resistance of the pellets was artificially raised from 750 Ω to match that of the Ag–AgCl electrodes. Calibration marks: 5 μV and 1 sec.

distribution and the electrode potential. Since the electrode potential of silver in a chloride medium is about 220,000 μV, it is apparent that minor changes in ion distribution easily could cause artifacts in an EEG range of 10-50 μV.

Such a system is also highly susceptible to steady currents through it. Steady currents polarize electrodes because as electrons enter tissue from an electrode they combine with positive ions such as hydrogen. Hydrogen atoms form hydrogen gas, which accumulates as an insulating barrier around a negative electrode if the current density is high and the gas is not able to diffuse away rapidly. Around a positive electrode, films of chlorides and other negative ions can occur. Such polarized electrodes impede current flow, especially low-frequency current, producing severe distortion of bio-electric signals.

There are several common situations in which electrodes become polarized. One is the use of monopolar square-wave current as a physiologic stimulus. More severe polarization occurs when DC current is used to make lesions (Section III, D). An often unsuspected source of polarization, especially in implanted electrodes with small surface area, is the use of ohm meters to check interelectrode resistance. These meters register resistance by passing DC current through the electrodes. If resistance must be checked *in vivo*, it should not be measured across a pair of implanted electrodes but between a large reference electrode on the mucosa or under the skin and each implanted electrode in turn, with implanted electrodes being negative (see also Chapter 3, Sections II and IV). Although all electrodes become charged by this procedure, there is not so much interelectrode polarization as when resistance is measured across pairs of electrodes.

B. NONPOLARIZABLE ELECTRODES

From the above, it should be clear that problems would be minimized if a silver electrode were placed in a solution with a high and stable concentration of silver, such as silver chloride solution. In practice, this situation is approximated by electrolytically coating a metal electrode with its poorly soluble salt, such as silver coated with silver chloride. In such a system, changes in silver ion distribution from the electrode would have much less effect on changing the overall ion concentration in the electrode region because the electrode is coated with a relatively large and stable concentration of silver and the chloride ion with which it reacts.

If current flows in one direction through such an electrode, silver ions move into the insoluble coat, and with reverse current they move into the electrode. Thus, the overall system remains relatively unchanged in the presence of current flow of either direction. Another major advantage of chlorided silver is that impedance for slow frequencies is approximately one-fifth that of unchlorided silver (Geddes and Baker, 1967).

There are several techniques for chloriding electrodes, but all have certain features in common. The basic principle is to pass electrons through pure silver immersed in sodium chloride solution. This forms hydrogen gas bubbles around the negative electrode, which also attracts sodium ions. The electrode connected to the positive pole of the battery attracts chlorine ions, and if that electrode is made of silver, the chlorine reacts to form a silver chloride coating upon the electrode.

The technique usually requires a 1½ V battery as the current source. The electrodes to be chlorided are scrubbed clean with sandpaper; metal brushes should not be used because they would contaminate the electrode with iron ions. Several electrodes can be connected in parallel to the positive pole, so that chloriding of each occurs simultaneously in a 5% sodium chloride solution. Current density should be low, of the order of about 2.5 mA/cm^2, in order to produce chlorided electrodes of low resistance and uniform coating. This requires chloriding to be done over relatively long periods, at least overnight. After chloriding, given pairs of electrodes show persistent potential differences that may amount to tens of millivolts or more. One worker has reported a more refined technique for chloriding that produces electrodes with an inter-electrode bias of less than 0.5 mV (Feder, 1963). Shorting the electrodes during storage discharges most of this bias potential. However, the bias gradually returns when the electrodes are in use. This slow drift is not important in AC recording but can be quite a problem in DC recording. If DC records are to be made, the electrodes should be stored open-circuited, or even with resistances added equivalent to the input impedance of the recorder. Then, drifting during recording will be greatly reduced. The initial steady potential difference can be canceled by DC balance circuits in the recorder.

Chloriding should be done in relative darkness, because the system is affected by light. When the electrodes are examined in light, proper chloriding is indicated by a uniform gray appearance caused by light reaction upon the AgCl coating. Exposure to light should be minimal, because bright light tends to reduce the chloride film and also to induce spike potentials that can appear as artifacts in the EEG (Fig. 2-2). Effectiveness of chloriding can be tested directly by connecting 2 chlorided electrodes to a 1½ V battery with an ammeter in series. When the electrodes are dipped into 1% sodium chloride, the current flow will be steady through properly chlorided electrodes. Improper chloriding will

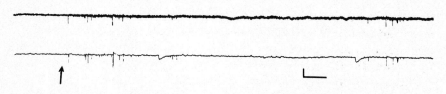

Fig. 2-2. Influence of bright light upon silver–silver chloride electrodes. Spikes were generated when room lights were turned on (arrow). The top trace is a recording between 2 conventionally chlorided electrodes placed in electrode paste, and the bottom trace is recorded between 2 chlorided pellet electrodes. Calibration marks: 5 μV and 1 sec.

be manifest by a sudden drop in current, indicating that polarization has occurred. Electrodes should be kept moist at all times by storage in saline. They also must be kept in relative darkness and be handled carefully to avoid scratching of the surface.

Although the chloriding procedure may seem a lot of trouble, properly prepared electrodes are usually stable for a week or more. Moreover, establishing a routine greatly simplifies the process.

A recent invention that may become widely used is the silver–silver chloride pellet electrode.[1] The pellets are made by mixing powdered silver and powdered silver chloride to form a solid, but somewhat porous, pellet under mechanical pressure. These pellets are more or less permanently stable and do not require any special preparation or maintenance by the investigator. The pellets have a very large effective surface area, and the metallic silver is kept in intimate contact with silver chloride to provide a very stable chemical junction. Another feature is the low DC bias voltage between electrodes, which is usually less than a few hundred microvolts.

Chlorided silver electrodes minimize, but do not eliminate, the problem of motion artifacts. Another aid is to use "salt bridges," such as electrode paste, between the tissue and the electrode. Various mechanical means can be devised to attenuate the magnitude of motion. In addition, placing the electrode in a baffle arrangement reduces the amount of movement that occurs in the electrode paste (refer also to Section II, A, and Chapter 3, Section VI).

All the foregoing discussion about chloriding does not apply to metal electrodes that are implanted in the brain itself because chlorided electrodes are toxic to tissue (Fischer *et al.*, 1961). The typical approach is to implant metals that are not very reactive, that is, do not dissociate readily, such as platinum, palladium, and various alloys of "noble" metals.

---

[1]Beckman Instrument Company, Palo Alto, California; Industrial/Medical Instruments, Newport Beach, California; In Vivo Metric Systems, Los Angeles, California.

C. Performance of Various Metals

Electrodes of various metals do not necessarily reproduce the same waveforms the same way. This is because the electrode–tissue interface is always associated with capacity and resistance due to chemical change during current flow, as shown in the equivalent circuit of Fig. 2-3. These 2 parameters depend on the character of the electrode chemistry and largely determine which frequencies appear across the amplifier input resistance (R_3) for subsequent amplification. Both C_1 and C_2 shunt higher frequency biopotentials away from the input resistance, because their resistance (reactance) to current decreases as the signal frequency increases, according to the formula

$$X_c = \frac{1}{2 f C}$$

where X_c is capacitative reactance, f is frequency in cycles per second, and C is the capacity in farads.

Shunting is especially serious in microelectrode studies of action po-

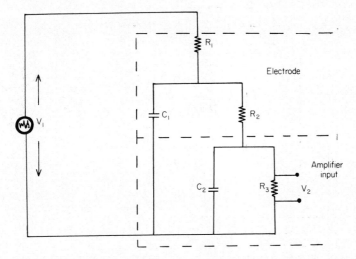

Fig. 2-3. Electrical equivalent circuit for an animal, electrodes, and amplifier input. Voltage from the animal (V_1) is applied via an electrode to the input resistance (R_3) of the amplifier where the signal (V_2) is passed on to amplifier stages. R_1 is the resistance due to the electrode in contact with electrode jelly and tissue fluids. R_2 is the resistance due to chemical changes occurring during current flow. The voltage across R_3 is directly related to the amplified voltage which appears at the pens of an EEG machine. C_1 is the capacitance caused by the electrode, and C_2 is that caused by wiring in the input circuit. The ratio of resistances between parallel capacitor and resistor routes determines which frequencies will be most faithfully amplified and which will be shunted away from the input resistance R_3 and will not be amplified.

tentials that have very high-frequency components. This problem is only solved with negative capacity amplifiers and cathode followers (Chapter 4, Sections I, A and I, B). Electrode conditions that create large capacity will increase the total input capacity and excessively shunt high frequencies away from the input resistance. In recording the typical EEG, either with surface or implanted electrodes, the factors most likely to increase capacitance are large electrode size and chemical reactivity of the electrode. Larger sizes create larger capacity, and increased reactivity causes more electrode ionization and charge separation at the electrode–tissue interface.[2]

Equally important as electrode capacity is the value of R_2, the resistance due to chemical reaction during current flow. For example, in nonpolarizable electrodes R_2 is very small, effectively shorting C_1 and shunting slow and DC potentials through the input resistance for faithful amplification. Conversely, highly reactive and polarizable electrodes would not record slow frequencies faithfully.

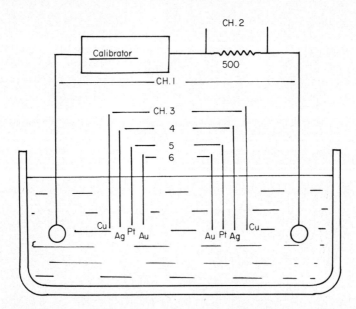

FIG. 2-4.   Technique for testing recording characteristics of various electrode metals. The calibrator drives a voltage through a saline, and that voltage is monitored on channel 1 (Ch. 1). Channel 2 monitors current by measuring voltage across a known resistance. (Cooper, 1963.)

[2]A method for testing the reactivity of any metal has been devised by Clarke and Hickman (1953). They published a list of commonly used electrode metals in a relative ranking of reactivity.

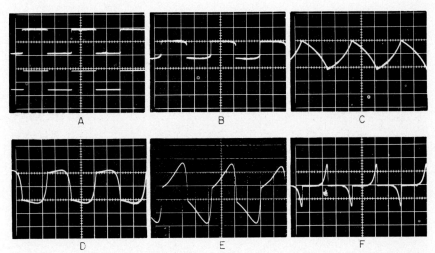

FIG. 2-5.   Qualitative comparison of recordings of square waves by various electrode materials. A: Driving waveform—the upper trace represents the voltage across the calomel–agar–calomel cell and the lower curve represents the current through this cell; B: recorded waveform from silver–silver chloride electrodes; C: carbon electrodes; D: platinum–10 iridium electrodes; E: stainless steel electrodes; and F: gold electrodes. (Roth *et al.*, 1966.)

The net effect of the interrelated variables upon the ratio of C_1, C_2, and R_2 is difficult to predict quantitatively, and for practical purposes it is simpler to test the electrodes for their reproducing properties. This is done by driving square waves from a calibrator through electrodes in physiologic saline solution and by observing the current waveform thus created by the various electrode pairs under study (Fig. 2-4). Sample results from such a procedure are shown in Fig. 2-5 and illustrate considerable distortion produced by the various electrode materials. However, more realistic appraisal might be possible if the driving current, instead of square waves, were sinusoidal in the frequency range of biological interest.

II. Affixing Surface Electrodes

A. Scalp Electrodes and Their Application

A suitable metal can be attached to tissue, such as the scalp, in such ways as inserting needle electrodes[3] under the skin or by clamping on miniature alligator clips. However, such methods do not take advantage

[3]Grass Instrument Company, Quincy, Massachusetts.

of an electrode-paste bridge, and the electrodes are highly susceptible to movement and artifacts. Tests of platinum subdermal electrodes revealed that they were relatively noisy and prone to produce motion artifact (Klemm, 1968a). They are, however, probably suitable for recording from anesthetized subjects that have higher EEG voltages and have no voluntary movements.

The ideal approach for scalp electrodes is to place a chlorided silver disk electrode on electrode paste that has been applied to the scalp. Proper preparation of the scalp requires clipping of excess hair and thorough cleaning of skin with alcohol. Where conditions permit, such as in anesthetized animals, scraping the skin with a scalpel blade to produce a "brush burn" establishes excellent conductivity. The electrode paste[3] does not have to be rubbed in, but merely placed upon the prepared spot of skin. To record from discrete points of skin, only discrete points of skin should be prepared and covered with electrode paste. It is also obviously important to avoid electric shorts resulting from confluence of paste from adjacent electrode sites.

The plain silver disk electrode[3] is not suitable for moving subjects but can be satisfactory for EEG studies in anesthetized animals. With electrode paste, the electrode needs no mounting but merely requires imbedding in the paste, which is sufficiently adhesive to hold the electrode. The paste tends to dry out, but usually remains satisfactory for at least 30 min. In conscious humans, collodion or Balsa cement commonly hold disk electrodes in place.

Disk electrodes can be "homemade," but the solder joints and lead wires require thorough insulation to prevent contact with electrode paste or tissue; otherwise, the different metals would generate transients in electrode potential.

The other type of scalp electrode illustrated (Fig. 2-6) has several advantages that make it the type of choice in moving animals. First, transparent tape with adhesive on both sides firmly attaches the electrode to the scalp (collodion is probably a better adhesive for hairy areas). When in place, the outer electrode shell surrounds the electrode paste, not only preventing drying but also reducing shifting of paste. Thus, whenever skin moves, the electrode moves, and there is little *relative* motion. Artifacts are produced by relative motion between the tissue or conductive paste and the electrode. Still further improvements are provided by additional baffling inside the outer shell of the electrode body. This is part of the inherent construction of the Beckman electrode. In the case of the Physiograph electrode, such baffling is easily provided by inserting a shirt button inside the shell of the electrode body. A removable baffle is necessary for the Physiograph type of electrode in order to permit

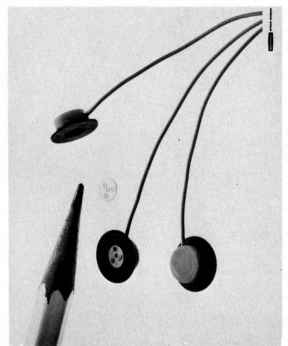

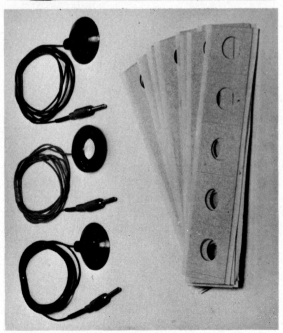

Fig. 2-6. Commercially available scalp electrodes. The silver electrodes on the left are produced by the E&M Instrument Company, Houston, Texas. Similar electrodes are available from Specialized Laboratory Equipment, Surrey, England, and from Becton-Dickinson, Westwood, Massachusetts. The silver-silver chloride pellets on the right are available from the Beckman Instrument Company, Palo Alto, California; other sources of such electrodes are listed in the footnote on page 38.

periodic cleaning and rechloriding of the silver disk. Although the Physiograph type of electrode lacks the merits of a pellet silver–silver chloride electrode, it has the advantage of being considerably cheaper. Other manufacturers[4] make similar self-adhering disk electrodes, but they are less amenable to chloriding.

Scalp electrodes someday may be made of electrically conducting silicone rubber. Such electrodes would have greater advantages of flexibility, moldability, ease of application, and less maintenance requirements. Although not yet perfected, one silicone rubber material seems especially promising (Jenkner, 1967).

B. SKULL ELECTRODES AND SURGICAL PROCEDURES

A much more satisfactory way to obtain surface EEGs from animals is to surgically install electrodes in the skull or on the cortex. [Refer to Delgado (1961) and Bureš *et al.* (1967) for reviews of various methods.] The electrode, especially when in bone, can be electrically insulated from most moving tissue fluids, avoiding artifacts from that source. Also, insulation from muscle greatly reduces problems with muscle potential artifact.

For most purposes the placement of electrodes on the dura or cortical surface seems to have no particular advantages and has the disadvantage that there is likely to be trauma and motion artifact due to vascular pulsations in meninges and brain. In any event, surgery requires the animal to be anesthetized or to be tranquilized and injected with local anesthetic in the incision region. Standard aseptic surgical precautions are required, although with certain laboratory species such as the rat and rabbit, these do not appear to be as critical as in animals such as the dog.

Aseptic procedure is a little difficult to obtain when the surgery is being done by one person, as is often the case. The author's routine approach, used successfully on rats, rabbits, cats, and goats, is not recommended to those who are not yet disciplined in the techniques of aseptic surgery, because surgery is done without surgical gloves and with only chemical sterilization. A major reason for this approach is that autoclaving and sterile surgery are not feasible because too many septic objects (drill, animal, bottles of cement reagents, etc.) have to be touched. Discipline and experience are necessary to control touching of objects that come into direct contact with tissue, thus increasing the likelihood of

[4]Telectrode, Telemedics, Inc., Southampton, Pennsylvania; Honeywell Corporation, Denver, Colorado.

infection. In no case do the hands touch tissue. Instruments are stored in a beaker of alcohol, with the handles up out of the solution. Before each instrument is used, it is shaken vigorously to rid it of excess alcohol. Residual alcohol does not hurt the tissues, and in fact there is evidence that it helps wound healing (Klemm, 1967) in addition to the antiseptic action. It is important, however, to keep alcohol away from any holes that have been drilled in the skull, as alcohol kills nervous tissue. After a given instrument is used, it is returned to the beaker of alcohol. Bleeding is controlled by electrocautery and by grasping sterile cotton with a forceps and sponging the tissue; bone wax is rarely needed.

Observations of students reveal that for some strange, perhaps psychological reason, they tend to be timid when cutting over the scalp. The incision, usually made along the saggital plane, should be made firmly in one strong stroke, of sufficient length to ensure adequate exposure of the skull. When electrodes are to be implanted over many skull regions, the cut should extend at least from between the eyes all the way back to the occiput. Although it is obvious, many investigators do not appreciate the fact that incisions do not heal lengthwise but heal from edge to edge; length of incision has little bearing on healing properties. After skull exposure, the entire observable periosteum is vigorously scraped away with the scalpel blade. This is essential to get good gripping by the dental cement[5] which is used later to anchor electrodes. The next step is to drill small skull holes to receive the electrodes. Drilling can be accomplished with a dental drill,[6] or more cheaply by a hand drill or by a small electric motor and flexible shaft.[7] Very few people have the required degree of touch control to prevent a sudden plunge of the drill when the skull is penetrated; as a result, considerable damage to meningeal vessels and cortical tissue occurs. The solution is to construct a stop on the drill but so that it can only penetrate to a certain preset depth; one of the simplest ways to do this is to put a ball of dental cement on the drill bit a few millimeters away from the tip.

There are many types of electrodes that can be implanted in this way; one of the first types used was a victrola needle hammered into the hole. Another approach is to cut short lengths of stainless steel hypodermic tubing, which are pressed into the hole. Another convenient method is to make electrode sets in a prearranged pattern. The whole set is subsequently fixed to the skull at one time (Fig. 2-7), as in the technique of DeVos and Bonta (1964).

[5]Grip Cement, L. D. Caulk Company, Milford, Delaware.
[6]C. H. Stoelting Company, Chicago, Illinois.
[7]Lafayette Radio Electronics, Syosset, New York.

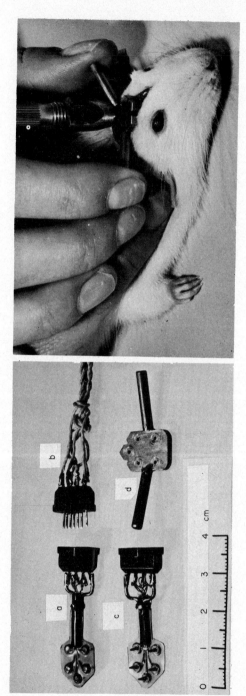

FIG. 2-7. Illustration on the left indicates one method for making electrode sets for insertion through the skull. a: Electrode set (upper side); b: connecting terminal; c: electrode set (under side); and d: guideplate for drilling skull holes. Picture on the right illustrates the method for drilling holes in the skull. (DeVos and Bonta, 1964.)

Miniature screws, made of stainless steel,[8] can be screwed in; these have the advantage of serving both as electrodes and as anchors for the dental cement. They have the disadvantage of creating connection problems. They may be grabbed with miniature alligator clips, but this is not always feasible because of limited space and motion of the contact junction. One can solder lead wires from a connector to the screws, but such soldering is not especially convenient. One could machine the screw so that it serves as a connector, receiving a spring type of plug, but this also is not convenient. There is a screw available[9] that has a knobbed end and a matching snap-on connector; although the screw is relatively large, it does provide a convenient method under some circumstances (Macchetelli and Montanarelli, 1965).

The author's own preference is to use insulated electrode wire (refer to Section III) that is bared at the tip and jammed horizontally into the trabeculae of the skull bone; the holes and wires are then covered with dental cement and the wires are soldered or crimped to a connector, which is likewise later embedded in cement.

It is important to place at least 2 anchoring screws if screws were not used as electrodes. The skull surface should also be as dry as possible for good adhesion of dental cement, a condition that is not always possible because of oozing blood. The cement should be made rather thick, so that it hardens rapidly before oozing blood can build up underneath it and prevent gripping of the skull. If oozing is excessive, electrocautery or bone wax will stop it.

Insertion of anchoring screws is sometimes difficult, requiring a hole of just the right size and firm gripping of the screw as it is being turned with a jeweler's screwdriver. The latter problem is greatly minimized by use of special self-gripping screwdrivers.[10]

Rats and cats may present special problems, because they will sometimes actively try to remove an electrode-connector assembly from their head by pulling on it with their feet and by trying to catch it in cage wiring. Such problems can be reduced by anchoring screws in the lateral skull surface instead of the dorsal (Goldstein, 1967). Rivets that can be mounted from one side; so-called "POP" rivets[11] are also effective (Roth, 1966). Inasmuch as these rivets are stainless steel, they also can be used

---

[8]J.I. Morris Company, Southbridge, Massachusetts; Small Parts, Inc., Miami, Florida; All-Stainless, Inc., Allston, Massachusetts; Elco Company, Rockford, Illinois; Star Stainless Screw Company, Patterson, New Jersey.

[9]Nu Way snap studs and fasteners, Allied Electronics, Chicago, Illinois.

[10]Ullman Devices Company, Ridgefield, Connecticut.

[11]Fastener Division, United Shoe Machinery Company, Shelton, Connecticut.

as electrodes, and they have a hollow shaft that could serve as a female connector. Another, very effective, approach (Phillips and Bradley, 1966) is to file the head of an anchoring bolt into a rectangular shape, drill a slightly larger rectangular hole in the skull, and insert the head end of the bolt until the head is just under the skull; then a 90° rotation of the bolt and placement of a nut on top of the skull will anchor the bolt. The bolts used by Phillips and Bradley were actually those on the connector they used, which was placed back on the bolts after they were in place. The bolts thus served to hold cement to the skull and also to hold the connector to the skull.

Techniques for closure of the operative site vary considerably, depending mainly on whether all electrodes are joined to a central, multi-contact connector. With a central connector, all exposed wires and joints are covered with dental cement and the skin is closed snugly around the base of the connector with nonabsorbing and nonabsorbable suture or steel clips.[12] If electrodes are dispersed and each serves as a connector, closure of the skin often is not feasible. Sometimes the incision can be sutured, followed by small incisions over each individual electrode-connector; care must be taken to ensure that cement insulates the electrode shaft from adjacent skin. If the incision can not be sutured, 2 or 3 loose suture ties are placed and dental cement is used to imbed the whole area, electrodes, skull, suture anchors, and incision edges. The anchor sutures prevent the incision edges from being pulled out from under the cement, which otherwise would expose them to bacterial contamination. Dental cement apparently does not seriously damage exposed flesh, and in fact it probably has considerable antiseptic action.

As a final step in the surgery, antibiotics, such as long-acting benzathine penicillin, are injected intramuscularly.

Although the surgical procedure seems involved, experienced workers can easily perform the entire operation in 30–45 min, which in the long run is a good investment of time for long-term EEG studies.

III. Implantation of Intracerebral Electrodes

A. Construction of Macro- and Microelectrodes

Macroelectrodes for depth implantation are made very readily.[13] The usual technique is to stretch small wire into straight pieces ready for

---

[12]Autoclips, Clay-Adams, Inc., New York, New York.

[13]In Vivo Metric Company, Los Angeles, California; Laboratory Concepts Company, New York, New York.

implantation; heating the wire under tension may be necessary. Wires need to be insulated with epoxy or varnish. The tip that will serve as the electrode can be scraped free of insulation (usually ½–1 mm). Wires need to be made of relatively nonreactive metal to improve recording fidelity and to reduce tissue damage.

In a histologic study of different implanted materials (Fischer *et al.*, 1961), silver–silver chloride produced inflammatory lesions approximately 1.5 mm in diameter within a week that did not change significantly during 4 weeks. Copper produced lesions of approximately 2.5 mm in diameter. Stainless steel (18-8) produced virtually no tissue reaction. All of the insulation materials tested produced no adverse effect.[14] Teflon has also been reported to be nontoxic in extracerebral tissue (Usher and Wallace, 1958).

Wire electrode size is important. Wire must be very small to minimize trauma, but the wire must be large enough to insert through brain tissue without bending. Usually, the ideal wire size is 30–34 gauge. Small, flexible wires can be inserted through a hypodermic needle cannula. Table 2-1 illustrates the current system in use for sizing electric wire.

A variety of small-gauge wire is commercially available. Many of these come conveniently coated with insulation, requiring the user only to bare the tip. Table 2-2 lists some of the types of wire available commercially.

Wire electrodes can be placed singly in various brain areas, in which case they would be used for "reference" recording (Chapter 5). In case "bipolar" recording is desired, electrode wires are inserted in pairs, either inside a hypodermic needle or twisted together. Paired electrode

TABLE 2-1
WIRE SIZES – GAUGE AND DECIMAL EQUIVALENTS

B & S Gauge	Inches	B & S Gauge	Inches
50	0.001	35	0.0055
49	0.0011	33	0.007
47	0.0014	32	0.008
44	0.002	31	0.009
42	0.0025	30	0.010
41	0.0028	29	0.011
40	0.0031	28	0.013
39	0.0035	27	0.014
38	0.004	26	0.016
37	0.0045	25	0.018
36	0.005	24	0.020

[14] Formvar, Beldon Company, Chicago, Illinois; Thermobond M-472, Sterling Varnish Company, Haysville, Pennsylvania; Tygon, U.S. Stoneware Company, Chicago, Illinois.

TABLE 2-2
SOME COMMERCIALLY AVAILABLE MONOFILAMENT WIRE SUITABLE FOR
INTRACEREBRAL ELECTRODES

Metal	Minimum gauge	Insulation	Supplier

Platinum
Platinum–
  rhodium
Platinum–
  tungsten
Chromel
Stainless steel
	38	Polyurethan, formvar
		silicone, etc.
			Consolidated Reactive
			Metals
			Mamaroneck, New York

Nichrome	30	Formvar	Driver-Harris Company Harrison, New Jersey
Platinum Platinum– iridium Palladium	50 40 50		Englehard Industries Newark, New Jersey
Tungsten	30		General Electric Cleveland, Ohio
Platinum– iridium	38	Teflon	Medwire Company Mt. Vernon, New York
Platinum Platinum– iridium Monel Stainless steel	36		Nessor Alloy Company Caldwell, New Jersey
Platinum Silver Gold	50	Oleoresinous, Isonell, modified silicone	Secon Metals White Plains, New York

tips are generally separated from each other by 1–2 mm vertically. Paired electrodes need checking to ensure that there are no shorts between them or with a hypodermic needle cannula; to prevent polarization, interelectrode resistance should be checked in air, not in tissue.

Both single and paired electrodes need checking also to ensure that there are no breaks in the insulation. This is most conveniently done by connecting a 1½ V battery to a pool of saline, in which the electrode to be tested connects to the negative pole and regular connecting wire is connected to the positive pole. Hydrogen gas bubbles will appear around the bared electrode tip and should not be present anywhere else along the insulated shaft. A dark background behind the saline facilitates observation. This check must not be made between 2 electrodes that will be implanted because they will polarize immediately.

Such wire electrodes can be made in various ways into multiple-contact electrodes. Multiple-contact electrodes have many advantages in that fewer skull holes are needed, surgery is easier, stereotaxic control is simplified, and localization is enhanced. Less brain damage is produced if the electrode assembly is made of very flexible wire and is implanted via a canula that is then withdrawn. The simplest way to make multicontact electrodes is to cut the number of wires required, bare the tip of each one, separate tips vertically as desired, and wrap the bundle with another piece of tightly wound wire. One can also form a bundle, grab each end with forceps, and twist the ends in opposite directions, maintaining a steady longitudinal pull. The degree of twisting should be enough to form a relatively tight bundle, but not so much as to prevent sliding some wires past each other to achieve spacing. Wires are spaced by pulling individual wires at one end. The electrode tips are then individually unraveled for scraping away insulation, followed by retwisting between the fingers. Tips must be formed smoothly, so that they do not project out from the bundle, which of course would greatly increase trauma during insertion. The "bubble" check previously mentioned will ascertain tip conductivity and reveal any insulation breaks.

A similar twisted-wire probe has been developed by Manning (1964). The technique requires the use of very small wire, annealed to be flexible. A bundle of electrode wires is wrapped with an extra wire that spirals around the bundle. At each point where a contact is desired, the extra wire is wrapped in closer spirals immediately above and below the desired contact area. Next, one of the wires is pulled out between the tight spirals, bared of insulation, and wrapped several times around the bundle. This technique has the advantage of ease of spacing and exposing individual contacts, as well as providing a radially non-selective contact area because the contact is exposed for 360° around the probe. However, the technique does not work well for 30–34 gauge wire and wire that is not specially annealed for flexibility.

Another, more sophisticated, technique for making multiple-contact intracerebral electrodes has been developed by Ray (1966).[15] This electrode features 18 separate wires laminated around a hypodermic needle; the overall diameter is less than 1 mm (Fig. 2-8).

Microelectrodes, by definition, are those with very small tip diameters, on the order of ½–10 μ. The small size contributes to a very high re-

---

[15] Advanced Systems Development Division, IBM Company, Rochester, Minnesota.

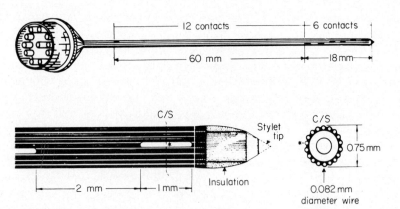

FIG. 2-8. Diagram of multicontact intracerebral electrode. The hollow stainless steel tubing stock core can be seen. Tips of the wires, cut off at the end, are insulated as shown. By cutting through the enamel of the wire at a selected point (*), a contact is established. Contacts may be cut anywhere along each wire. Probe contact spacing used is shown. (Ray, 1966.)

sistance, ranging from 1 to 40 megohm in tissue. The high resistance features require special electronic coupling to an EEG amplifier, which is discussed in Chapter 4. By virtue of their small size, microelectrodes record from a very small volume of tissue and can be used for intracellular recording.

Construction of microelectrodes,[16] a tedious process, can be achieved. with electrolyte-filled glass tubes or electrolytically sharpened wire. The glass type usually exhibits better performance characteristics, but it is not popular for chronic implantation in brain, unless DC potentials must be recorded.

Glass electrodes are made by mechanically pulling heated glass tubing (1–7 mm diameter Pyrex) into a fine tapered point (Bureš *et al.*, 1967; Bilanow, 1967). The electrolyte filler for the tubing is usually 3.5 *M* KCl for intracellular recording or concentrated NaCl for extracellular recording. Filling is achieved by submerging electrodes in an airtight vessel of electrolyte solution. The solution is heated to boiling and the steam is sucked out by a vacuum pump. As the electrodes fill, small bubbles appear at the large open end. Although filled electrodes can be stored a short time, the time is limited by formation of salt crystals. Refer also to the papers by Bennett (1956) and Kao (1954).

Metal microelectrodes are made by electrolytically etching small-gauge

[16]Transidyne General Corporation, Ann Arbor, Michigan.

wire (36–40 gauge). In the techniques of Hubel (1957) and Green (1958), alternating current of about 7 V is supplied to the electrode, the tip of which is submerged in 10–20% HCl. The other pole, also submerged in the acid, is a carbon rod or silver foil. To prevent splattering of acid, a layer of xylol is floated on top. During current flow, the electrode is raised up and down to produce a tapering point. Near the end of the process, voltage is decreased to improve the quality of the point. When finished, the electrode is dipped in strong $NaCO_3$ solution, then in 1% acetic acid, and then in xylene. While still wet with xylene, the electrodes are insulated by dipping in thick lacquer[17] for 30 sec. After quick withdrawal, electrodes are inverted vertically and allowed to air dry at room temperature for several hours; they are then baked overnight at 60°C. Surface tension and gravity prevent insulation from covering the extreme tip of the electrode. The quality of the insulation is checked with the "bubble" check referred to previously for macroelectrodes. This check is not possible if electrodes are very small—less than 1 μ.

There is some disagreement over which metal is best for microelectrodes. Bureš *et al.* (1967) prefer tungsten because it is not as brittle as stainless steel. On the other hand, Green (1958) prefers stainless steel because it is less noisy, is easier to straighten, and permits localization by the Prussian blue technique (Section III, D).

Kinnard and MacLean (1967) have developed a technique for making platinum microelectrodes that feature relatively low resistance and noise. A piece of 70% platinum–30% iridium is straightened by heating under slight tension. Dipping 10–15 times in a solution of 50% NaCN and 30% NaOH to which 5–6 V AC is applied etches the tip to a few microns; current is decreased for final polishing of the tip. Successive dips in water, toluene, and ether clean the electrode.

Prior to insulation, the electrode is coated with platinum black to decrease resistance. The electrode is connected in series with a 1 megohm resistor to the negative terminal of a 1.5-V battery and is lowered 15–25 μ into a 1% solution of platinum chloride while current is passed for 2–3 sec. To insulate, the wire is placed with its tip upward in a device for lowering it into unthinned paint (Dupont 828-014 gray paint). The electrode is dipped by a motor-driven micromanipulator at a speed of 0.65 mm/sec until all but 0.5 mm of the tip is immersed. Then the manipulator is hand operated to lower all but 40 μ of the tip. At this point, the motor is reversed and wire is raised at the same speed

[17]Insl-X E33, Insl-X Company, Yonkers, New York.

as during lowering. After air drying under a beaker for 20 min, the electrode is baked for 20 min at 380°F.

The next step is testing with a capacitance meter according to the method of Bak (1967) for detection of breaks in insulation and estimation of uninsulated tip length. If after a second coat the capacity is greater than 20 pF and the uninsulated tip more than 30 μ, the paint is applied to within 20 μ of the tip. Two to four coats may be required to obtain satisfactory insulation and a desired tip capacitance of 5–15 pF.

The finished electrode includes a protective implantation shank (Fig. 2-9) made of 28-gauge hypodermic tubing, which is electrolytically polished at both ends. A similarly polished piece of 22-gauge tubing serves as a guide and protective covering for the microelectrode as it is lowered into tissue.

All the techniques so far discussed are very time-consuming. As one remedy, Mills (1962) has proposed a relatively mass-production means of making microelectrodes. By this method one can make 20 micro-electrodes within an hour of working time. Pieces of electrode wire are separated from each other by about 2–4 mm and soldered at right angles to the axis of a rod, as shown in Fig. 2-10. A glass container is filled with equal parts of H_2SO_4, H_3PO_4, and water. A 2-cm² piece of platinum serves as a cathode in the solution. The rod is mounted in a sleeve at each end so that it rotates parallel to the liquid, dipping electrodes through on each revolution. One end of the rod is connected to a 24-V DC motor by a short piece of plastic tubing for flexibility. A

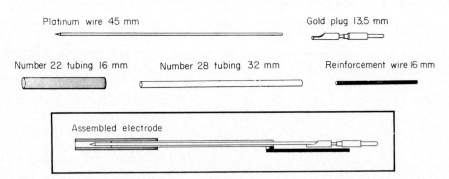

FIG. 2-9. Platinum microelectrode; components of the electrode are illustrated. Electrode is ensheathed in a guide that protects the tip and directs its course after insertion in the brain. (Kinnard and MacLean, 1967.)

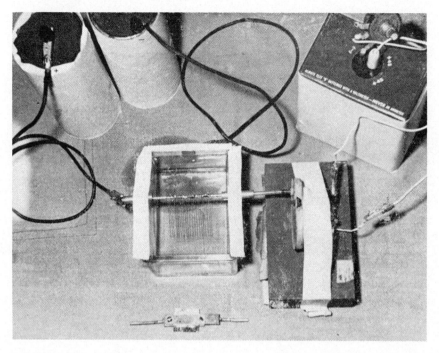

Fig. 2-10. Equipment setup for relative mass production of microelectrodes. (Mills, 1962.)

potentiometer of about 5 kilohm is connected in series with a 45-V battery, and the motor then is adjusted to give a rotation rate to the rod and wires of about 5 rpm. The wire is connected to the anode of a battery (3 V) at the sleeve in which the rod rotates. Every half hour the direction of rotation is reversed; over a period of 6 hr tips become etched to diameters of 1-6 μ. Mills' technique for insulation involves use of Formvar; the tip is dipped and slowly withdrawn with a micromanipulator. Electrodes are mounted vertically with tips upright and baked for 30 min at 150°C; dipping and baking are repeated 4 times. Of the electrodes finished in this way, 60-75% will have a tip diameter of 1-6 μ.

Essentially the same method can be used for tungsten wire, except that the electrolyte solution is changed to 0.5 M NaOH and wires are mounted in a clamp for rotation (tungsten does not solder well and requires spot welding).

B. Surgery and Use of the Stereotaxic Atlas

The surgery required for implantation of intracerebral electrodes is basically similar to that previously described (Section II, B). The major differences are determination of skull burr-hole sites and the actual implantation of electrodes.

Accurate electrode placement depends upon stereotaxic techniques. Such techniques involve a mapping of the brain in 3 planes, so that one can predictably implant an electrode in any part. The basic idea of a stereotaxic map can be demonstrated with a few illustrations from the atlas of the rabbit brain (Monnier and Gangloff, 1961; Fig. 2-11). These diagrams illustrate how the brain can be mapped in sagittal, coronal, and horizontal planes. A basic reference point is needed from which these maps are constructed, and in most cases this reference point is the bregma.[18] Anterior–posterior and lateral measurements from the bregma, when correlated with the stereotaxic atlas, permit drilling of skull burr holes that lie directly over the intended region of implantation. The atlas also provides the necessary information on how deep the electrode must be inserted to reach the implant region.

Stereotaxic atlases for many species have been published. Among these are atlases for the guinea pig (Hoffman, 1957; Liberson and Akert, 1955), the rabbit (Fifková and Maršala, 1967; McBride and Klemm, 1969; Monnier and Gangloff, 1961; Sawyer et al., 1964), the rat (Fifková and Maršala, 1967; DeGroot, 1959; Massopust, 1961; Pellegrino and Cushman, 1967; Snider and Niemer, 1961), the sheep and goat (Andersson, 1951), the cat (Bleier, 1961; Fifková and Maršala, 1967; Desmedt and Franken, 1958; Jasper and Ajmone-Marsan, 1961), the dog (Adrianov and Merink, 1959; Lim and Liu, 1960), and the monkey (Olszewski, 1952; Russell, 1961). In the event an atlas is not available for the species of interest, the investigator must make his own. A relatively simple procedure is outlined by Fifková and Maršala (1967).

Measurement of the required distances on the skull can be done quite simply with a millimeter rule. After burr holes are drilled, electrodes

---

[18]The intersection of sagittal and coronal sutures.

Fig. 2-11.   Illustration of the basic idea of a stereotaxic map. Top picture is a stained sagittal section, 1.5 mm from the midline, of a rabbit brain. Ao, area occipitalis; Apa, area paracentralis; Apc, area praecentralis; Apop, area praeoptica; Cb, cerebellum; CA, cornu ammonis; Coi, colliculus inferior; Cos, colliculus superior; CFo, columna fornicis; Ca, commissura anterior; Cp, commissura posterior; CC, corpus callosum; CMm, corpus

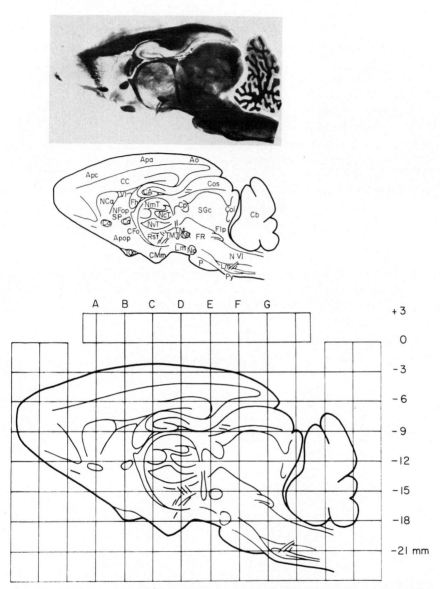

mamillare mediale; Flp, fasciculus longitudinalis posterior; Fh, fimbria hippocampi; FR, formatio reticularis; Lm, lemniscus medialis; N VI, nervus abducens; NCa, nucleus caudatus; NcT, nucleus centralis thalami; NFop, nucleus fornicis proprius; Nip, nucleus interpeduncularis; NmT, nucleus medialis thalami; NR, nucleus ruber; NvT, nucleus ventralis thalami; P, pons; Py, pyramis; Rst, regio subthalamica; SP, septum pellucidum; SGc, substantia grisea centralis; TMT, tractus mamillo-thalamicus; TM, tractus Meynert; TOp, tractus opticus; Vl, ventriculus lateralis. The bottom diagram shows the dimensions among various regions in the brain; all grids are 3-mm square. (Monnier and Gangloff, 1961.)

should be inserted in the same vertical plane as that prescribed by the atlas. This can be achieved most simply by attaching an electrode guide block on the skull in such a way that it overlies the burr holes and assures perpendicularity of electrode insertion. A simple technique of this sort, actually a modification of the method of Monnier and Gangloff (1961), has been published (Klemm, 1964). The first step is to make a lucite guide block that can be screwed to the skull (Fig. 2-12). The block is oriented over burr holes, electrodes are inserted to the proper depth, dental cement is poured around the base of the electrodes, and the block is removed.

In lieu of some type of guide block attached to the skull, the usual approach (Fig. 2-13) involves the use of an elaborate stereotaxic apparatus.[19] The basic features of these units are that they have a holder to keep the head in proper planes and electrode holders that move predictably in all required planes. Such devices have the advantage of being very accurate but have the disadvantage of being expensive. Each electrode must be cemented in place before another can be implanted.

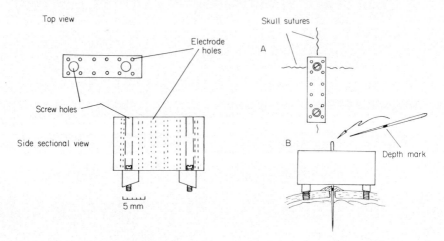

Fig. 2-12.   Illustration of a simplified method for stereotaxic implantation of electrodes in brain. On the left is a scale drawing of the plexiglass block; the block is temporarily fixed to the skull as a guide for inserting electrodes, as shown in the illustrations at the right. The block is oriented over skull sutures, with the bregma as a reference point (A). The side sectional view shows electrode insertion and fixation with dental cement, after which the guide block is removed (B). (Klemm, 1964.)

[19] Baltimore Instrument Company, Baltimore, Maryland; Kopf Instruments, Tujunga, California; Lehigh Valley Electronics, Fogelsville, Pennsylvania; Narishige Instrument Company, Farmingdale, New York; Neuman and Company, Skokie, Illinois; Pfeiffer Company, Old Lyme, Connecticut; Stoelting Company, Chicago, Illinois.

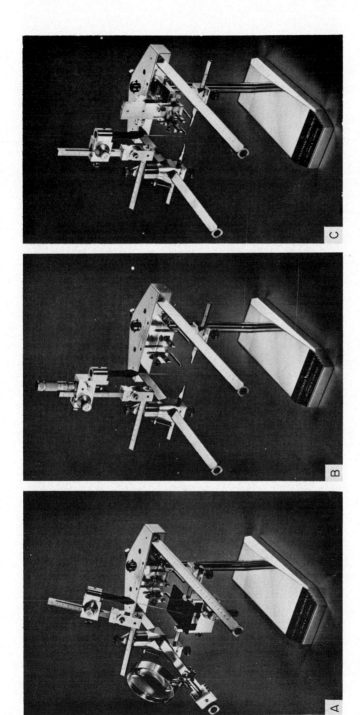

FIG. 2–13. Stereotaxic instrument. A: L-101 Electrode locating grid with magnifier; B: M-102 electrode carrier with micrometer drive; C: G-105V fixation attachment arranged for squirrel monkeys. (Courtesy of H. Neuman and Company, Skokie, Illinois.)

59

When many electrodes are being implanted, the process can be quite slow and the bulk of cement material can be excessive. Ray (1965) has devised a simply constructed plastic skull cap, which, when screwed on the skull, serves to hold each implanted electrode while successive ones are being implanted.

A homemade and inexpensive apparatus has been developed by modifying a microscope, which should be suitable for very small laboratory animals such as the rat (Barry *et al.*, 1963). Another device has been developed that employs a milling table (Bull and Collins, 1966). An example of another homemade device is shown in Fig. 2-14.

Where multiple-contact electrodes are to be inserted into one burr hole, stereotaxis is greatly simplified. Depending on the degree of accuracy required, the electrode assembly can be inserted free hand in an anesthetized animal through a guide tube, such as hypodermic tubing, which has been previously anchored in the burr hole.

Electrodes whose depth can be adjusted after implantation are very convenient because they permit exploration of many brain areas with only one initial operation. The technique of Long and Tapp (1965) permits adjusting the depth over a 4.5-mm range. Electrodes are fixed inside a nylon screw that turns inside a nut that is mounted to the skull. The alignment of the electrode wires inside the screw is critical, because lack of perpendicularity will cause the electrode to rotate in a circle when turned, increasing brain damage.

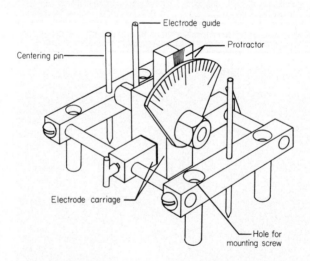

FIG. 2-14. Homemade stereotaxic device, originally devised for head mounting on pigs. (Courtesy of O. F. Roesel, School of Veterinary Medicine, Purdue University, Lafayette, Indiana.)

A simple, ingenious device for adjustable implantation of gross electrodes has been developed by Schmidt (1969). This concept was employed in designing the device illustrated in Fig. 2-15 (Klemm, 1968b). The electrode carrier is threaded to move up and down on a captive bolt. Turning of the movable bolt causes the electrode carrier to move up and down. Among the special features of this unit are a millimeter scale, capacity to hold several electrodes, and anchoring screws that permit ready removal of the whole unit for reuse. With the unit anchored to the skull, electrodes are inserted to the desired depth through a guide tube and are then anchored to the movable electrode carrier that has been set at its lowest point. During recording the electrode is moved dorsally, and when full excursion is reached the electrodes can be anchored at the top plate, released from the movable carrier, and reanchored to the movable carrier after it has been lowered. Releasing the top anchor allows another complete excursion.

Adjustability is still more valuable with microelectrode studies in chronic preparations, because activity from many individual neurons should be sampled. A number of techniques have been developed (Davis and Tollow, 1966; Evarts, 1968; Hayward *et al.*, 1964; MacLean, 1967; Oomura *et al.*, 1967).

C. Affixing Electrodes to Connectors

Connectors are necessary for both scalp and intracerebral electrodes. In the case of scalp electrodes, lead wires are usually plugged into pin jacks, which in turn are soldered to the amplifier input. Most EEG recorder manufacturers supply electrode plug-in boards with their units; such boards also can be easily, and less expensively, made by the investigator. Intracerebral electrodes are usually best connected by soldering to a connector that is mounted on the head; the connector in turn mates with another connector and lead cable that plugs into pin jacks in an electrode board.

Connectors are an important link between electrodes and the input receptacles of amplifiers. Many times connectors are the weakest link in the chain of components, being a possible source of high resistance and motion artifact. Ideally, all junctions should be soldered; in acute, one-time experiments electrodes can be soldered directly to lead wires. In animals prepared for chronic studies, however, soldering lead wire to the electrodes requires bundling all the lead wires in a package on the animal; this is inconvenient for the investigator and the animal may tear at the package of wires. The usual solution is to solder electrodes to a connector mounted on the head, which during an experiment is mated to a cable of lead wires.

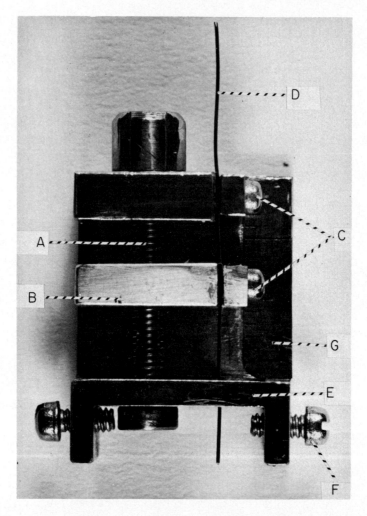

Fɪɢ. 2-15.   Adjustable macroelectrode implanting device. A: Captive bolt with knob at top for turning, which causes the electrode carrier plate (B) to move up or down; B: electrode carrier plate; C: electrode anchor screws – top screw is normally left loose to allow free vertical movement of electrodes; D: electrode wire, anchored at electrode carrier plate (B) and passing through hole in base (E) for insertion into brain; F: base anchor screws that are tightened around wire arms that protrude from unit for imbedding in dental cement; G: millimeter rule. (Klemm, 1968b.)

Connectors are usually joined to the electrode and connecting wires by melting solder, an alloy of tin and lead, around the joint. Soldering can be difficult, especially with most poorly reactive metals used as intracerebral electrodes. Some metals, like tungsten, may require spot welding. The general principles of soldering have been reviewed by

Luke (1961). Usually the parts to be soldered are first coated with flux, which removes oxide films and improves the quality of the soldered junction. Flux, as well as solder itself, should be applied only to the parts being heated, not the soldering iron. Whenever possible, only the noncorrosive resin flux should be used. However, many alloys used as electrodes do not solder properly with resin flux and require special fluxes such as concentrated zinc chloride solution.[20]

A solder joint is more durable if good mechanical contact is provided before soldering. In addition, the parts being soldered must be made quite hot prior to application of solder. Do not move the soldered joint until it is cool. A good indication of the quality of a solder joint is the color when cool; it should be shiny and not dull.

One of the biggest problems in soldering, especially with poorly solderable metals, is the buildup of residues on the soldering iron. Soldering irons, especially when they are overheated, become rapidly coated with combustion debris that prevent good soldering. Overheating can be reduced by interposing a variable transformer between the iron and the wall socket. It is often necessary to scrape combustion residue off with a sharp object between each junction soldered. The scraping should be done as the iron cools after heating, until the iron is shiny when cool. Melting solder directly on the tip and scraping assists in this process, known also as "tinning." The need for proper tinning cannot be overemphasized, because most poorly reactive metals will not otherwise be solderable.

After a connector is soldered to implanted electrodes, it might be tempting to test the resistances between each pin to determine the presence of any shorts from the solder flux. However, this would polarize the electrodes and therefore is not advisable. This is an argument for presoldering and checking all electrodes *before* they are implanted; yet this is not always feasible. To check for high resistances due to incomplete soldering, the testing should be done outside the body or, with implanted electrodes, it should be done between one implanted electrode and a hypodermic needle stuck under the skin; polarity of the electrodes should be negative.

In some cases it may be desirable to use conductive cement around the junctions.[21] Such cement will create an electrically conductive junction with any metal, and it usually must air dry for several hours.

It may be more convenient to spot weld noble metals than to solder

---

[20] Special flux and solder—Wescolite Kit—for poorly solderable metals is available from Caig Laboratories, New Hyde Park, New York.

[21] Number 1777 conductive cement, Electrofilm, Inc., Cherry Hill, New Jersey.

them. One handy welding device[22] is available that is so precise that it can throw a flame of 6300°F through the eye of a needle.

The simplest form of connector is a miniature alligator clip that can be clamped on the electrodes. This is most satisfactory if the electrode is relatively large and has a rough surface, as with screw electrodes. However, alligator clips have two serious disadvantages: their relatively large size and their tendency to move around the electrode shaft. They are definitely not suitable for conscious, moving animals.

Similar comments could be made about jewelers clips or other slip-on contacts, which can be clamped over smooth-shaft electrode terminals. Such terminals are readily made by cutting short pieces of hypodermic needle tubing, grinding the ends, and crimping one end over the electrode wire.

Because most studies require simultaneous connection of many electrodes, miniature, multicontact connectors are commonly preferred. They can be conveniently mounted in cement on the head, ready at any time for connection to a cable. Many types of suitable connectors are available commercially.[23]

The major advantage of such connectors, their close spacing of contacts, is also the major disadvantage, inasmuch as soldering is tedious. Special care is needed to prevent solder or flux on adjacent pins from touching; after soldering interpin resistances must be checked. Another cumbersome feature of most connectors is that wires cannot be mechanically fastened before soldering. Most connectors are relatively expensive, and it often is desirable to devise anchoring brackets from which dental cement can be broken away to allow reuse of the connector.

The heat conduction during soldering of small implanted wires is insufficient to produce demonstrable brain damage. If larger wires are used, a "heat sink" using a hemostat placed on the wire near the solder point may be used.

What is really needed is a better selection of nonsolderable connectors. One such device is the Sheatz pedestal, with 8 or 10 contacts, which is commercially available,[24] but is relatively expensive (Sheatz, 1961). For some applications, screw-type terminal strips may be satisfactory.[25] For

[22] Tescom Company, Minneapolis, Minnesota.

[23] Amphenol Connector Division, Chicago, Illinois; Continental Connector Corporation, Woodside, New York; Elco Corporation, Willow Grove, Pennsylvania; ITT Cannon Electric, Los Angeles, California; National Connector Corporation, Minneapolis, Minnesota; Winchester Electronics, Oakville, Connecticut.

[24] Laboratory Concepts, Inc., New York, New York.

[25] Cinch Company, Chicago, Illinois; Kulka Company, Mount Vernon, New York; and National Tel-tronics Company, Yonkers, New York.

most purposes, however, crimp-contact connectors with removable contacts would be preferable.[26]

Construction of the cable that will be used in connecting the animal to the recorder must be done carefully. Each solder joint must be tested to assure good conductivity; likewise, each connection point must be checked against the others for shorts that might have been created by careless soldering or excessive flow of flux. Finally, the electrostatic shields around each conductor in the cable all must be connected together and tied to a ground lead; conduction in the shield system must be checked, and shorts must be checked for between the shield and each conductor. Shield-conductor shorts are very likely when making cables from the special low-noise wire[27]; the insulation separating the shield and conductor has a conductive film on it which must be scraped off in the region of the exposed conductor tip.

The finished cable then should be checked for "cross talk" between wires, since current flowing in one wire can capacitatively induce current in an adjacent wire. The simplest method is to deliver a signal of the largest voltage expected in any experiment to one pair of leads in the cable. The 2 cable wires closest to those carrying current should be connected to a resistance equivalent to animal impedance and recorded from simultaneously with the main signal channel. Such tests indicate that individually shielded wires in a cable are much less likely to exhibit cross talk.

D. LOCALIZATION OF IMPLANTS

Checking electrode placement after experimentation is an essential procedure because of inherent anatomic variability. An extensive review of this subject has been written by Akert and Welker (1961).

At the end of an experiment, electrode sites are usually marked in some way to become more evident during gross or microscopic examination. The most common method is to electrolytically destroy tissue by passing DC current through the electrodes. A voltage source of about 30 V or more is used to pass the current, which must be continuously monitored by an ammeter. Current flow is regulated by a series potentiometer, and one usually can expect lesion size to be about 1 mm of diameter per minute that each 1 mA of current is passed. In the case of "monopolar" electrode arrangements, anodal lesions are preferable to cathodal, since during electrolysis less gas is formed at the anode; thus mechanical tissue distortion is less, and the shape of the lesion is more regular.

[26] Amphenol Company, Chicago, Illinois; the 220 series contacts and the 9-pin Tiny Tim connector are especially useful and economical.

[27] "Mini-Noise" Coaxial Cables, Microdot, Inc., South Pasadena, California.

It may be necessary to keep an animal alive for several days after making such lesions, because the area of dead tissue will be more evident then. Lesions of about 1 mm or more are easily detected grossly when brain slices of about 1 mm are made; in some circumstances, this may be all that is needed for verification of electrode position.

Gross observation of gray and white matter is facilitated by gross staining of the brain by the LeMasurier technique (1935), which stains gray matter blue and leaves white matter unchanged. A similarly useful stain is Snider's toluidine blue method (1943), which also stains gray matter blue against a nearly colorless background.

Should better definition of electrode position be required, there are other site-marking techniques. Often one simply makes a very small lesion with direct current, or, if the brain were well fixed with electrodes in place, sections in the proper plane will reveal the tract where electrodes had been. If the electrodes used contain iron, as in stainless steel, the reaction of ferrous iron with potassium ferricyanide can be used to mark the electrode site. In this technique about 4 V of DC is passed through the electrodes for 10 sec (Longo, 1962). The resulting deposit of metal from the electrode can be stained bright blue by immersing the fresh whole brain for 48 hr in a solution composed of 15 parts of potassium ferricyanide, 150 parts of formalin, 750 parts of alcohol, and 1300 parts of distilled water. Conventional histologic techniques are then used to process the brain.

In the case of marking sites of microelectrode tips, the technique of Henriques and Sperling (1966) should be useful (Fig. 2-16). This method deposits free iron ions iontophoretically through the glass microelectrode that was used for recording. The iron is subsequently stained with a Gomori stain.

Before one can localize the position of intracerebral electrodes, either grossly or microscopically, the brain must be properly fixed in formalin. If swelling is not a problem, best results are obtained with 25% formalin, instead of the usual 10%. The best procedure involves bleeding of the animal while still alive, under surgical planes of anesthesia, followed by a brief period of flushing the brain arteries with water, followed by perfusion with formalin. Once the animal is anesthetized, the sternum is cut rapidly with heavy bone shears (or wire cutters); the right auricle is slashed, the aorta is clamped, and the perfusion needle is inserted into the left ventricle. Alternatively, one can sever the jugular veins and perfuse through the carotids with a ligature placed behind the point of entry of the perfusion needle. Within a few seconds water should be gravity fed into the left ventricle (or carotids) until the effluent from the jugular veins is clear, followed immediately by formalin perfusion. As formalin reaches the brain, distinct body movements will occur and

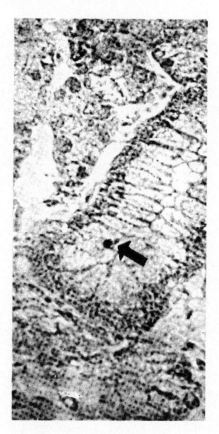

Fig. 2-16. Marked ductular cell of the submaxillary gland in which iron ions had been electrophoretically deposited from a glass microelectrode in order to mark the electrode's location (arrow). (Henriques and Sperling, 1966.)

persist for some time. Often the heart will continue beating for several seconds while pumping formalin; should the heart stop at any time, flow is assured by gravity and can be assisted by manual pumping of the heart.

It is best to slowly perfuse the brain for an hour or more with electrodes still in place. Then, when electrodes are removed, they will be more likely to leave a definite identifying hole and will be less likely to destroy adjacent structures during removal.

In some situations an animal may die before perfusion can be performed, especially when electrolytic lesions are made in crucial areas and the animal is sustained for several days to allow the lesions to develop. In these situations the whole head must be soaked in formalin for several days. The brain must be exposed so that formalin can diffuse in; this is best achieved by clearing away tissue from the base of the skull and by sawing a coronal section across the nose just in front of the brain.

When the brain is properly fixed, the next step is to remove it. Skin should be freed from anchoring sutures and dental cement, anchoring screws should be removed, and the electrode-cement assembly should be carefully removed in the same approximate plane as that of original insertion.

Removal of electrodes from perfused brain is not difficult if electrodes were implanted vertically. Removal of anchoring screws and slight jiggling will free the cement; a quick vertical pull will remove electrodes without excessive tearing of tissue. However, if electrodes have been implanted at severe angles, it may sometimes be necessary to dissect out the electrodes by careful breaking away of bone and cement.

Before breaking away the skull bones, the zero reference point in the brain needs to be marked, either by a large needle or by a razor blade inserted in the same plane in which electrodes were implanted. For gross brain slices, a manipulator or stereotaxic electrode holder can be used to make slices in the proper plane.

The most convenient way to remove skull bones is to saw out a hole over a region of unimportance with a rotary saw attachment for flexible drill shafts. Then a pair of forceps can be used to break away bone from the brain until the brain is exposed, whereupon the brain can be scooped out.

If histologic sections are to be made, the brain first must be cut into a block that contains area of electrode placement. Ideally, the histologic sections should be in the same plane as the electrodes, a feat that is not easily accomplished. Reference needles can be inserted stereotaxically in the same plane as the electrodes; the block of tissue then can be cut in the same plane as the reference needles. Rocha-Miranda *et al.* (1965) have developed a stereotaxically oriented macrotome for precise cutting of blocks of brain tissue (Fig. 2-17). Richer (1968) has devised a simpler way to block the brain without reusing the stereotaxic device; he removes the brain and simply lays it on an incline which, when the brain is cut vertically (90°), will be the equivalent plane to that obtained by use of the stereotaxic device.

In many cases there is no great need for cutting tissue in the exact plane of electrode insertion. Where electrode tracks are visible, some workers deliberately slice off the plane of insertion. Examination of serial sections reveals a hole that appears successively lower in successive sections; location of the last hole marks the site of the electrode tip. Where electrolytic lesions have been placed at the electrode tip, it may not be necessary to slice brain in the plane of electrode insertion.

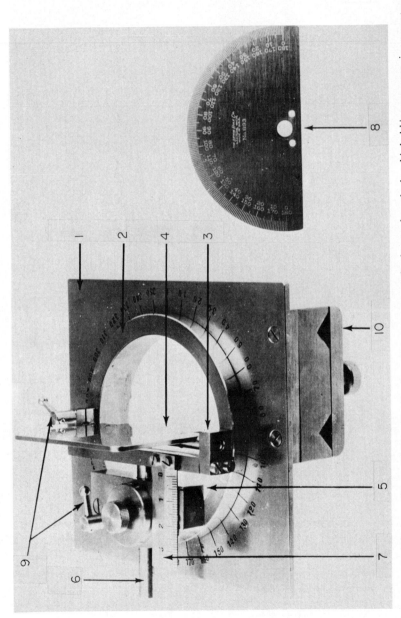

FIG. 2-17. Macrotome for cutting blocks of brain tissue in exact stereotaxic planes when the head is held in a stereotaxic apparatus. Base plate, (1), upon which rests a rotating ring, (2). Mounted on the ring is the carriage, (3), for the sectioning plate, (4), which is used to guide the plane of sectioning—position of sectioning plate is adjusted by moving the pin, (6), in the undercarriage, (5). Tilt of sectioning plane can be adjusted and measured by a protractor, (8), which mounts on the carriage—tilt adjustments are held by set screws, (9). Support under base plate, (10), is used to clamp device to ear bars of stereotaxic apparatus. (Rocha-Miranda *et al.*, 1965.)

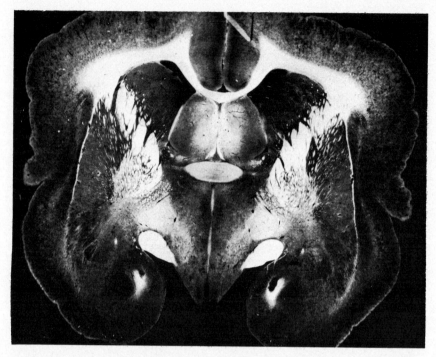

FIG. 2-18. Photograph of formalin-fixed, unstained frozen section of rabbit brain. Slide was placed in an ordinary photographic enlarger and used as if it were a negative.

Histologic examination of the brain should follow standard procedures. The usual stains include hematoxyline-eosin or, for more precision, the Weil or Weigert stains for myelin or the Nissl stain for cells. One staining technique recently has been described that allows staining of unimbedded, frozen sections (Wolf and Yen, 1968).

There are several rapid histologic methods available, all based on the use of frozen sections. The technique of Guzman *et al.* (1958) involves formalin perfusion of the brain with electrodes *in situ*, followed by freeze-microtome sections of 150–200 μ. All sections that show the electrode tract are mounted directly from water on a glass slide and dried with blotting paper. Sections are then put into a photographic enlarger, and a photographic print is made. Similar techniques of photographing the projected image from fresh and wet unstained sections have been reported by Powell (1964), Hutchinson and Renfrew (1967), and Siegel (1968). In our laboratory best results have been obtained with 90 μ sections, cut at −20° C, and floated in water on a slide. Exposure parameters were 5–15 sec at F 8; high contrast print paper, Kodabromide F 5 (McBride and Klemm, 1968). An unretouched sample photograph is illustrated in Fig. 2-18. We have prepared a complete rabbit brain atlas which shows the actual photographs of the tranverse sections at 1 mm intervals.

A final method of electrode localization should be mentioned: the measurement of electric impedance changes in various regions of the brain (Robinson, 1962). Although this method is very unconventional, the accuracy is better than that of conventional stereotaxic approaches because placements are made in accordance with neural rather than cranial landmarks, the distance of electrodes from known points is therefore much shortened, and cumulative or consistent stereotaxic errors are negated. The method is especially useful because it permits confirmation of electrode position *during* implantation and thus allows any necessary correction before experiments are begun. Robinson, who used a Wheatstone bridge to measure impedance, showed that different brain regions of monkeys exhibited sufficiently distinct impedance values to distinguish them. Differences were especially marked between extracranial fluids, neuronal areas, and fiber tracts.

REFERENCES

Adrianov, O. S., and Merink, T. A. (1959). "Atlas Mozga Sobaki." Medgiz, Moscow.

Akert, K., and Welker, W. I. (1961). Problems and methods of anatomical localization. *In* "Electrical Stimulation of the Brain" (D. E. Sheer, ed.), pp. 251–260. Univ. of Texas Press, Austin, Texas.

Andersson, B. (1951). The effect and localization of electrical stimulation of certain parts of the brain stem in sheep and goats. *Acta Physiol. Scand.* **23**, 8–24.

Bak, A. F. (1967). Testing metal micro-electrodes. *Electroencephalog. Clin. Neurophysiol.* **22**, 186–187.

Barry, T. J., Hagamen, W. D., and Sherlock, J. E. (1963). Microscope as a stereotaxic instrument for the rat. *J. Appl. Physiol.* **18**, 445–446.

Bennett, M. V. L. (1956). The response of cerebral cortex and adjacent tissues to stimulation of somatic sense organs and their nerve fibers. Thesis, University of Oxford, Great Britain.

Bilanow, G. (1967). Micro-pipette pullers: Some detail and technology. *Electroencephalog. Clin. Neurophysiol.* **23**, 376–378.

Bleier, R. (1961). "The Hypothalamus of the Cat." Johns Hopkins Press, Baltimore, Maryland.

Bull, J. A., and Collins, T. B. (1966). A homemade stereotaxis. *Am. J. Psychol.* **79**, 647–648.

Bures, J., Petráň, M., and Zachar, J., eds. (1967). "Electrophysiological Methods in Biological Research," 3rd rev. ed. Academic Press, New York.

Clarke, E. G. C., and Hickman, J. (1953). An investigation into the correlation between the electrical potentials of metals and their behavior in biological fluids. *J. Bone Joint Surg.* **35B**, 467–473.

Cooper, R. (1963). Electrodes. *Am. J. EEG Tech.* **3**, 91–101.

Davis, R., and Tollow, A. S. (1966). Adjustable stimulating and recording electrodes in brain of the unrestrained animal. A study of red nucleus. *Electroencephalog. Clin. Neurophysiol.* **21**, 196–200.

DeGroot, J. (1959). "The Rat Forebrain in Stereotaxic Coordinates." Noord-Hollandsche Uitgevers, Amsterdam.

Delgado, J. M. R. (1961). Chronic implantation of intracerebral electrodes in animals. *In* "Electrical Stimulation of the Brain" (D. E. Sheer, ed.), pp. 25–36. Univ. of Texas Press, Austin, Texas.

Desmedt, J. E., and Franken, L. (1958). Lesions experimentales dans l'encephale du chat: Methode et controles anatomiques. *Arch. Intern. Pharmacydyn.* **114**, 487–490.

DeVos, C. J., and Bonta, I. L. (1964). A simple permanent electrode set for tracing cortical electrograms in the rat. *Arch. Intern. Pharmacodyn.* **147**, 280–284.

Evarts, E. V. (1968). A technique for recording activity of subcortical neurons in moving animals. *Electroencephalog. Clin. Neurophysiol.* **24**, 83–86.

Feder, W. (1963). Silver-silver chloride electrode as a non-polarizable bioelectrode. *J. Appl. Physiol.* **18**, 397–401.

Fifková, E., and Maršala, J. (1967). Stereotaxic atlases for the cat, rabbit, and rat. *In* "Electrophysiological Methods in Biological Research" (J. Bureš, M. Petráň, and J. Zachar, eds.), pp. 653–731. Academic Press, New York.

Fischer, G., Sayre, G. P., and Bickford, R. G. (1961). Histological changes in the cat's brain after introduction of metallic and plastic-coated wire. *In* "Electrical Stimulation of the Brain" (D. E. Sheer, ed.), pp. 55–59. Univ. of Texas Press, Austin, Texas.

Geddes, L. A., and Baker, L. E. (1967). Chlorided silver electrodes. *Med. Res. Engr.* pp. 33–34.

Goldstein, R. (1967). A method to reduce dislodgement of implanted cranial electrodes in rats. *J. Exptl. Anal. Behav.* **10**, 290.

Green, J. D. (1958). A simple microelectrode for recording from the central nervous system. *Nature* **182**, 962.

Guzmán, C. F., Alcaraz, M. V., and Fernández, A. G. (1958). Rapid procedure to localize electrodes in experimental neurophysiology. *Bol. Inst. Estud. Med. Biol. Mex.* **16**, 29–31.

Hayward, J. N., Fairchild, M. D., Stuart, D. G., and Deemer, J. A. (1964). A stereotaxic platform for micro-electrode studies in chronic animals. *Electroencephalog. Clin. Neurophysiol.* **16**, 522–524.

Henriques, B. L., and Sperling, A. L. (1966). Marking of sited cells after electrophysiologic study. *J. Appl. Physiol.* **21**, 1247–1250.

Hoffman, G. (1957). "Atlas vom Hirnstamm des Meerschweinchesns." Hirzel, Leipzig.

Hubel, D. H. (1957). Tungsten microelectrodes for recording from single units. *Science* **125**, 549–550.

Hutchinson, R. R., and Renfrew, J. W. (1967). A simple histological technique for localizing electrode tracks and lesions within the brain. *J. Exptl. Anal. Behav.* **10**, 277–280.

Jasper, H. H., and Ajmone-Marsan, C. (1961). Stereotaxic Atlases. Diencephalon of the cat. *In* "Electrical Stimulation of the Brain" (D. E. Sheer, ed.), pp. 203–231. Univ. of Texas Press, Austin, Texas.

Jenkner, F. L. (1967). A new multi-purpose electrode material for general bio-medical application. Report to Dow Corning Center for Aid to Medical Research, Midland, Michigan.

Kao, C.-Y. (1954). A method for making prefilled microelectrodes. *Science* **119**, 846.

Kinnard, M. A., and MacLean, P. D. (1967). A platinum micro-electrode for intracerebral exploration with a chronically fixed stereotaxic device. *Electroencephalog. Clin. Neurophysiol.* **22**, 183–186.

Klemm, W. R. (1964). Simplified method for stereotaxic implantation of electrodes in brain. *Am. J. Vet. Res.* **25**, 1564–1565.

Klemm, W. R. (1967). Enhanced healing of skin wounds in dogs with systemically and locally administered drugs. *Experientia* **23**, 55–57.

Klemm, W. R. (1968a). Attempts to standardize veterinary electroencephalographic techniques. *Am. J. Vet. Res.* **29**, 1895–1900.

Klemm, W. R. (1968b). Adjustable macro-electrode implantation device for long-term EEG studies. *Comm. Behav. Biol.* **2**, 137–139.

LeMasurier, H. E. (1935). Simple method of staining macroscopic brain sections. *A.M.A. Arch. Neurol. Psychiat.* **34**, 1065–1067.

Liberson, W. T., and Akert, K. (1955). Hippocampal seizure states in guinea pigs. *Electroencephalog. Clin. Neurophysiol.* **7**, 211–222.

Lim, R. K. S., and Liu, C.-N. (1960). "A Stereotaxic Atlas of the Dog's Brain." C. Thomas, Springfield, Illinois.

Long, C. J., and Tapp, J. T. (1965). An inexpensive adjustable electrode for chronic implantation. *Electroencephalog. Clin. Neurophysiol.* **19**, 412–413.

Longo, V. G. (1962). "Rabbit Brain Research," Vol. II. Elsevier, Amsterdam.

Luke, R. W. (1961). Soldering. *Am. J. EEG Tech.* **1**, 112–119.

McBride, R. L., and Klemm, W. R. (1968). Stereotaxic atlas of rabbit brain, based on the rapid method of photography of frozen, unstained sections. *Commun. Behav. Biol.* **2**, 179–215.

Macchetelli, F. J., and Montanarelli, N., Jr. (1965). A simple chronic cortical electrode for the monkey. *J. Exptl. Anal. Behav.* **4**, 636–640.

MacLean, P. D. (1967). A chronically fixed stereotaxic device for intracerebral exploration with macro- and micro-electrodes. *Electroencephalog. Clin. Neurophysiol.* **22**, 180–182.

Manning, G. C., Jr. (1964). A new miniature multi-contact electrode for subcortical recording and stimulation. *Electroencephalog. Clin. Neurophysiol.* **17**, 204–208.

Massopust, L. C., Jr. (1961). Stereotaxic atlases, Diencephalon of the rat. *In* "Electrical Stimulation of the Brain (D. E. Sheer, ed.), pp. 182–202. Univ. of Texas Press, Austin, Texas.

Mills, L. W. (1962). A fast inexpensive method of producing large quantities of metallic microelectrodes. *Electroencephalog. Clin. Neurophysiol.* **14**, 278–279.

Monnier, M., and Gangloff, H. (1961). "Rabbit Brain Research," Vol. I. Elsevier, Amsterdam.

Olszewski, J. (1952). "The Thalmus of the Macaca Mulatta." Karger, Basel.

Oomura, Y., Ooyama, H., Naka, F., and Yamamoto, T. (1967). Microelectrode positioners for chronic animals. *Physiol. Behav.* **2**, 89–91.

Pellegrino, L. J., and Cushman, A. J. (1967). "A Stereotaxic Atlas of the Rat Brain." Appleton, New York.

Phillips, M. I., and Bradley, P. B. (1966). Micro-miniature connectors used as permanent electrode holders in the rat. *J. Exptl. Anal. Behav,* **9**, 291–292.

Powell, E. W. (1964). A rapid method of intracranial electrode localization using unstained frozen sections. *Electroencephalog. Clin. Neurophysiol.* **17**, 432–434.

Ray, C. D. (1965). Multiple electrode implantation in animals. A simplified plastic cap technique. *Electroencephalog. Clin. Neurophysiol.* **19**, 529–530.

Ray, C. D. (1966). A new multipurpose human brain depth probe. *J. Neurosurg.* **24**, 911–921.

Richer, C.-L. (1968). A simple device to orientate rat brain for cutting according to DeGroot's Atlas. *Proc. Soc. Exptl. Biol. Med.* **126**, 701–702.

Robinson, B. W. (1962). Localization of intracerebral electrodes. *Exptl. Neurol.* **6**, 201–223.

Rocha-Miranda, C. E., Oswaldo-Cruz, E., and Neyts, F. L. K. (1965). Stereotaxically oriented macrotome: A device for blocking the brain in rectangular and polar co-ordinates. *Electroencephalog. Clin. Neurophysiol.* **19**, 98–100.

Roth, J. G. (1966). A method for attaching apparatus to the skull. *Electroencephalog. Clin. Neurophysiol.* **20**, 618–619.

Roth, J. G., MacPherson, C. H., and Milstein, V. (1966). The use of carbon electrodes for chronic cortical recording. *Electroencephalog. Clin. Neurophysiol.* **21**, 611–615.

Russell, G. V. (1961). Stereotaxic atlases. Hypothalamic, preoptic, and septal regions of the monkey. *In* "Electrical Stimulation of the Brain" (D. E. Sheer, ed.), pp. 232–250. Univ. of Texas Press, Austin, Texas.

Sawyer, C. H., Everett, J. W., and Green, J. F. (1964). The rabbit diencephalon in stereo-taxic coordinates. *J. Comp. Neurol.* **101**, 801–824.

Schmidt, R. S. (1969). Preoptic activation of frog mating behavior. *Behaviour* (in press).

Sheatz, G. C. (1961). Electrode holders in chronic preparations. Multilead techniques for large and small animals. *In* "Electrical Stimulation of the Brain" (D. E. Sheer, ed.), pp. 45–50. Univ. of Texas Press, Austin, Texas.

Siegel, J. (1968). A rapid procedure for locating deep electrode placements. *Physiol. Behav.* **3**, 203–204.

Snider, R. S. (1943). A rapid bulk nissl method. *Stain Technol.* **18**, 35–39.

Snider, R. S., and Niemer, W. T. (1961). "A Stereotaxic Atlas of the Cat Brain." Univ. of Chicago Press, Chicago, Illinois.

Usher, F. C., and Wallace, S. A. (1958). Tissue reaction to plastics; a comparison of nylon, orlon, dacron,teflon, and marlex. *A.M.A. Arch. Surg.* **76**, 997–999.

Wolf, G., and Yen, J. S. (1968). Improved staining of unimbedded brain tissue. *Physiol. Behav.* **3**, 209–210.

3

Noise or Artifact

I. General Considerations

Noise, or artifact, means many things to many people. In electro-biology noise refers to unwanted electric potentials that are mixed with the bioelectric signal of interest. The amplitude of noise must be kept small, relative to the biologic signal; in other words, the signal-to-noise ratio should be as large as feasible.

Noise is probably the most common problem encountered by electro-encephalographers. Although they would not like to advertise the fact, most electrobiologists have inevitably had considerable experience with artifacts.

Noise can originate from many sources, those external to the animal and those within it. Noise from outside the animal quite often comes from the recording instrument and from electric power lines. In the animal, there are many different sources of electric noise, some of which are difficult to distinguish from EEG potentials.

This chapter is designed not only to discuss and illustrate various common types of artifacts, but also to present methods for reducing such artifact. The reader will find that although only experience can bring full appreciation of the problems, this chapter can greatly expedite the ability to recognize and deal with artifacts. Further detail can be found in the publications by Kay (1964), Nastuk (1964), Stacy (1960), Whitfield (1959), and Yanof (1965).

II. Source Noise

Much noise originates from the animal itself and the connections between it and the input of the amplifier. Recording from an electrode pair of dissimilar metals (Chapter 2, Section I, A) produces excessive noise due to fluctuating electrode potentials. Usually, source noise is associated with the resistances in the animal and amplifier input circuit. Random motion of electrons and ions, in the animal and in the wires, generates a broad frequency band of noise. When these small currents flow through large resistances, random voltages are developed that may be amplified sufficiently to appear in the EEG. In addition to random electron motion, there is induced electron motion and noise from nearby power lines (refer to Section IV).

The amount of noise that appears in the EEG also depends on the frequency band of the amplifier. For this reason, most EEG machines have filters that begin to attenuate signals at around 50 cps. Many have filters specifically designed to exclude the power line frequency of 60 Hz (cps). Rejection of all high frequencies is usually acceptable unless one wishes to study high frequencies or action potentials, in which case the noise level recorded inevitably increases. The mean square noise level $\overline{E^2}$, in addition to being proportional to resistances and bandwidth, is also proportional to absolute temperature. The overall relationship is expressed by Johnson's equation:

$$\overline{E^2} = 4\,R \cdot k \cdot T \cdot \Delta f = 1.6 \times 10^{-20} \ \text{V}^2/\text{cycle}/\Omega \ \text{at } 27°C$$

where E is the noise voltage, R is the resistance, k is the Boltzmann constant, and Δf the bandwidth in cycles per second. The rms voltage is obtained by taking the square root of $\overline{E^2}$; the peak-to-peak voltage equals about 2.8 times the rms value. A fairly typical example of bandwidth influence on noise level can be given by considering an intracellular recording situation wherein the resting MP and action potentials are being monitored. The bandwidth could possibly range from DC to 10 kc. Assuming an electrode impedance of 10 megohms, the rms noise level would be about 40 μV $(1.6 \times 10^{-20})(1 \times 10^4)(1 \times 10^7)$, and the peak-to-peak voltage would be about 112 μV. However, if the study were restricted to DC measurement with an upper frequency cutoff at 1 Hz, the noise level would be only about 1.1 μV, peak to peak. Similarly, reducing the impedance greatly reduces the noise. If we assume the original requirement of a 10 kc bandwidth but employ a 1 megohm impedance, the peak-to-peak noise voltage will be only about 35 μV.

Good electrode contact is essential to ensure an adequate signal-to-noise ratio. The quality of electrode contact can be measured by determining the electric resistance of the animal and its electrodes. When resistances are measured with an ohmmeter, the values obtained refer to DC resistance, and considerable error is involved because the DC current generated by the meter polarizes the electrodes (refer to Chapter 2, Section I, A). Although the values obtained are too high, for practical EEG purposes this is no problem. If in spite of this error interelectrode resistances are less than a few thousand ohms, the contacts are satisfactory for EEG recording.

A more accurate resistance measurement can be made with AC current; values of impedance obtained are only valid for the frequencies tested. A Wheatstone bridge is the conventional instrument used for such determinations. However, a much simpler method is available, although surprisingly it is not used often. The technique is based on "loading" the input. For example, assume that a high-impedance amplifier is monitoring an EEG that has peak voltages of 100 μV. If one connects a potentiometer in parallel with the animal impedance and adjusts the resistance until the peak EEG amplitude is only 50 μV, bioelectric current flow in the input circuit will be equally divided through the resistor and the animal. Thus the resistor value is equivalent to the impedance of the animal at the frequencies the animal is generating.

Another cause of source noise is resistance changes that result from jiggling motion of electric contacts in the input. Figure 3-1 illustrates

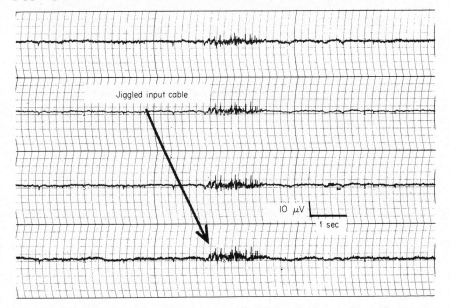

FIG. 3-1. Example of the artifacts produced by jiggling the input cable at the connection to the amplifiers.

such noise, which looks amazingly similar to an EEG. Note that although only 1 input cable was juggled, the artifact appeared in all channels. A comparable source of noise is a connector used on an animal with implanted electrodes; movement of lead wires often will cause movement of connector contacts, creating noise.

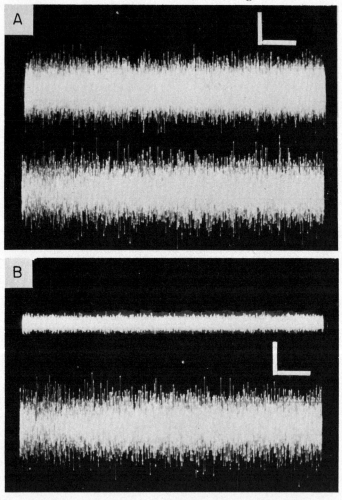

FIG. 3-2.   A: Comparison of electronic noise recorded with high gain (top oscilloscope trace) and multiple neuron action potentials recorded at lower gain (bottom trace). Calibrations: 5 μV (top trace) and 20 μV (bottom trace); 100 msec. B: Illustration of the principle of signal-to-noise ratio. Both traces recorded at same gain. Top trace is noise, obtained with no signal input and with amplifier connected across a 47,000-Ω resistor. Bottom trace was obtained from multiple neuron action potentials. Calibrations: 20 μV; 100 msec.

III. Instrument Noise

All electronic equipment generates noise due to random motion of electrons in the wires, tubes, and transistors. This noise is dependent upon the circuit and the nature of components used. For several years inherent transistor noise was much greater than that in electron tubes, and this prevented the use of transistors in EEG equipment. However, in more recent years, transistors have been developed with acceptably low noise levels.

The reader need not concern himself with design problems associated with noise (refer to Smullin and Haus, 1959). He need only take note of the overall noise level in his equipment. This noise level is usually stated in the manufacturer's specifications; the level should be about 1 μV, with the input leads shorted and well shielded. A more meaningful measure of noise, unfortunately seldom specified, is that present with a resistance between the input leads.

Noise from tubes and transistors in a recorder can become a special problem when one studies high-frequency phenomena such as nerve action potentials. This is less of a problem with EEG recording because the faster noise frequencies can be removed by electric filtration (Chapter 5, Section III, B, 3). Simultaneous recording of action potentials from numerous neurons can produce a tracing that looks very much like noise, especially if the gain of the recorder or monitoring oscilloscope is increased (Fig. 3-2A). To know for certain how much noise contributes to the trace, the signal-to-noise ratio can be determined by simultaneously recording noise and the signal at the same gain on separate channels (Fig. 3-2B). Noise level should be determined by replacing the animal with a resistor that approximates the animal's impedance.

IV. Electrostatic–Electromagnetic Interference

Electrostatic interference arises from the fact that an electrically charged body induces a separation of charges on a nearby conductor. Any conductor attached to a voltage source, whether or not it carries current, will generate an electric field that can induce charges on nearby conductors. This induction follows the law that like charges repel and unlike charges attract. An example of such induction is shown in Fig. 3-3A.

A conductor that has been polarized (charges separated) is usually unintentionally connected via the air to ground; these high resistance air paths nonetheless permit accumulated electrons to "leak off" to ground. This flow of electrons develops a voltage difference across that leakage resistance, which when sufficiently amplified is readily detectable, often to the point of obscuring other signals of interest. The scheme is depicted in Fig. 3-3B.

In most biologic recording situations, the source of interference is from power lines and wall sockets.[1] The character of this interference is mostly electromagnetic, in that power line currents set up an alternating magnetic field that in turn induces current in conductors connected to the amplifier inputs. The interference may still be present even if nothing is plugged into the wall sockets, i.e., no current is flowing. In this case, interference will be less but can still be excessive if the amplifier input is too close. The character of the interference from open wall sockets is electrostatic, in that wall sockets and conductors attached to the animal act like capacitor plates separated by an air dielectric. Inasmuch as power line voltage alternates and capacitors will alternately charge and discharge in response to the alternating voltage, an alternating charge can be induced on the animal (Fig. 3-3C). Noise is thus amplified along with the bioelectric signals. Sources of higher frequency electromagnetic interference include radio and television stations and some "intercom" systems.

When bioelectric signals are very small, on the order of less than 1 mV, interference becomes particularly objectionable and often completely obscures observation of bioelectric signals. One important way to minimize such interference is to increase the separation of the source and the animal. Induced voltage will decrease with increasing distances from the animal (Fig. 3-4). It also sometimes is helpful to disconnect all

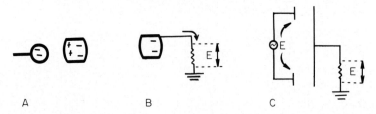

A   B   C

Fig. 3-3.   A: Electrostatic induction. An electrically charged body, when brought close enough to another conductive body, will induce a charge separation on that body. B: Development of interference voltage. As charge leaks off to ground through high resistance paths, a voltage is developed across those paths. C: Interference in bioelectric recording situations. Alternating current sources (shown at left) alternately induce voltages in the experimental preparation (symbolized on the right).

[1] 60 Hz in the United States; 50 Hz in many other countries.

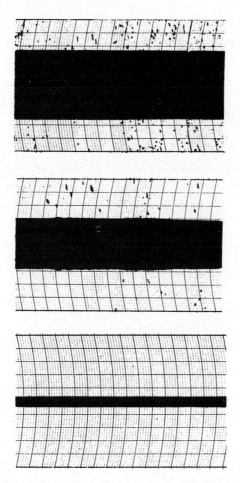

Fig. 3-4. Influence of distance on the magnitude of 60-cycle interference that is re-corded. Recordings were obtained from open-circuited probes placed 1, 2, and 3 ft (top-to-bottom traces) from an electric wall socket that was open-circuited.

unnecessary appliances and circuits. In cases where power lines of greater than 110 V are present, it may be impossible to avoid excessive interference, even when using the additional techniques mentioned below.

Another way to reduce the recording of interference is to keep the resistance between recording electrodes as low as possible. The higher the resistance, the greater will be the interference voltage developed across that resistance (Fig. 3-5). The most common cause of high interelectrode resistance is failure to ensure good electrode contact,

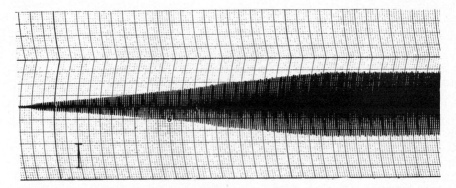

Fig. 3-5. Influence of interelectrode resistance upon magnitude of 60-cycle interference that is recorded. Resistance was increased from 0 to 5000 Ω (left to right). Calibration mark: 20 mV.

which in the case of skin electrodes often requires that the skin be defatted and even scraped with a scalpel blade until much of the epidermis is removed. Drying of electrode jelly will also cause high interelectrode resistance. Another cause is a break in the conducting wire, which often occurs at flection points in fine, stranded wire.

Even when all of the above precautions are taken, 60 Hz interference may still be present. In such cases it is necessary to surround the animal with a metallic shield, which when connected to ground will intercept the induced voltages and carry charge off to ground. The most satisfactory way to do this is to line the walls of an entire room with metal sheeting, connecting to ground at one point.[2] The room should be connected, at one point only, via a large conductor (at least 000 power bus) that is driven into the ground to a depth that is perpetually moist. This ground should be separate from that to which any other laboratory connects. Special care must be taken to shield the wall and light sockets and to ensure that no unshielded appliances or cables are in the room. Detailed construction procedures are provided in the publication by Thompson and Yarbrough (1967). This procedure is obviously expensive, and many investigators prefer to make a screen wire cage of appropriate size. Such cages can be very simple (stapled wire screen of 3/8-in. mesh or smaller over a wooden frame) or very elaborate (sound attenuated and temperature controlled; Lee, 1967). If ordinary window screen is used, individual strands may eventually corrode and

[2] Copper foil with self-adhering backing may be obtained from Sissalkraft Company, Carey, Illinois. Copper-coated plywood is available from U.S. Plywood Company, New York, New York.

poor electric contacts between strands may develop. Some newer types of screen are only loosely woven and therefore still less desirable. Galvanized screens, or "hardware cloth," are better because they are first woven and then dipped in molten metal; such processing produces better electric contact at each junction.

Because electrostatic interference can be propagated from all directions, the shielding cage must completely surround the animal, although occasionally one will find that a door of the cage can be left open to facilitate manipulations, especially if the cage is turned in certain directions. Commercial recorders and oscilloscopes need not be placed inside the shield because they usually have a built-in shield. There should be no pipes, wires, or other conductors inside the enclosure.

Grounding has many associated subtleties that may cause problems. Grounding of each item should occur only once, and all ground wires should be brought to the same point. This is more difficult to accomplish than it may seem. Many times interference persists in EEG recordings because the investigator has created "ground loops" in his placement of ground wires. In such ground loops, interfering current continues to circulate from equipment through ground and back to equipment. A common oversight is inattention to the grounding of the recorder. If the power cable to the recorder has a shielded cable and a 3-prong plug (and most do), the outer frame of the recorder is automatically grounded when the instrument is plugged into the wall socket (provided the socket is properly grounded). Therefore, ground loops are best avoided by bringing individual ground wires from the cage and elsewhere to a single point that connects directly with the chassis or ground connection of the recorder.[3] Examples of proper and improper grounding are illustrated in Fig. 3-6.

Although it is common to place a ground on the animal, such practice should be discouraged. Grounding an animal, when recording electrodes are connected to differential amplifiers, can reduce the grid-to-ground resistance in all channels, causing some interaction between channels (Bureš *et al.*, 1967). Many times it is necessary to ground an animal to reduce electric stimulation artifacts. In these cases the EEG should be recorded with and without ground to make certain there is no objectionable change in the essential character of the EEG in each channel.

---

[3]In some buildings the electric ground is inadequate. In such cases one can construct a ground with a long copper rod driven into the ground. Or a ground can be placed on water pipes, provided the resistance is less than a few ohms. Keep the ground wire as short as possible. Do not ground to gas pipes, compressed air or drainpipes.

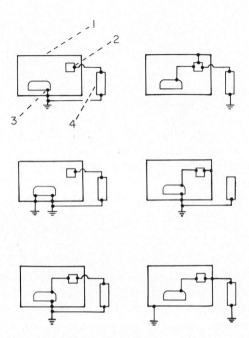

FIG. 3-6. Diagrammatic illustration of grounding methods for EEG apparatus. The upper 2 examples are correctly grounded, except ground wires on the preamplifier at the right should be at the same point. The lower 4 diagrams illustrate ground loops and incorrect grounding. Screen wire cage enclosing animal and preamplifier (1), preamplifier (2), animal (3), and recorder (4). (Klemm, 1965.)

Electromagnetic interference results from the magnetic fields generated by moving electrons in conductors. When these fields intersect other conductors, current is induced to flow. The situation is analagous to transformer coupling of electricity, where current flow in the primary induces a current in the secondary.

Grounding of such interference is more difficult than electrostatic shielding because more dense shielding material is required, such as iron or the alloy mumetal. Iron is quite cheap, but mumetal has much greater attenuating capability (Thompson and Yarbrough, 1967). A magnetic shield could also serve as an electrostatic shield when properly grounded. Such heavy shielding is not required for electrostatic shielding, and thus it is often simpler just to remove sources of electromagnetic interference from the recording area; electromagnetic field intensities decrease inversely as the square of the distance. If removal is not feasible, for example, when an electric motor is used in the experiment, the best solution is to shield the source.

A common though often unsuspected source of noise is electrode leads that move with respect to each other. Variation in capacitance between each lead, electrostatic charges on the insulation, and electro-magnetic effects of electron flow in the wire can all contribute to large artifacts and "cross talk" between leads. As seen in Fig. 3-7, the artifact voltages can be quite significant, especially if large amplification is needed to record the signal of interest. The figure also demonstrates that this problem is greatly minimized by shielding each wire[4]; induced currents are thus carried off to ground. Another way to attenuate these artifacts is to form the lead wires into a cable, which limits the amount of motion that occurs between leads.[5] Kamp *et al.* (1965) have described a technique for making a shielded, multiconnector cable that has a small diameter and a light weight. Cable noise can be still further reduced by use of special low-noise wire,[6] which is essential for use with freely moving animals.

The electroencephalographer who understands noise and its elimina-tion will still find it very useful to conduct a "dry run" with his equipment before connecting an animal into the circuit. This is best done by record-ing with amplifiers connected to a resistance substitution box or to a po-tentiometer. With the box and input leads properly shielded, the user should then dial in various high resistances, using high amplification, and determine if the noise level is acceptable. If the noise level is too high, that is, sufficient to distort the animal's bioelectric signals at the amplification setting that will be used, then the user can leisurely make necessary adjustments. If he discovers excessive noise only after an experiment is begun, matters can become quite frustrating and hectic. Inasmuch as most experiments create enough problems on their own, it seems prudent not to compound those problems by simultaneously trying to deal with excessive noise. After recording from a "resistor" proves satisfactory, the investigator can proceed with the experiment with some confidence.

Another preliminary check with the animal in the circuit is to check the resistance of each electrode to ensure good contact and low resis-tancetance. This can be done by connecting an ohmmeter to a known low-resistance contact (for example, a hypodermic needle under the skin or an electrode likely to have good contact) and switching in each elec-trode to be examined. If such facilities are not built in the recorder, the simple circuit in Fig. 3-8 can be used. The unit can be made easily by mounting a rotary switch and appropriately connected input jacks.

[4]Sources of such wire are the Birnbach Radio Company, New York, New York, and Calmont Company, Santa Ana, California.
[5]Several companies supply small wire cables with variable numbers of conductors. One such source is the Spectra Strip Wire Company, Garden Grove, California.
[6]"Mini-Noise" coaxial cables, Microdot, Inc., South Pasadena, California.

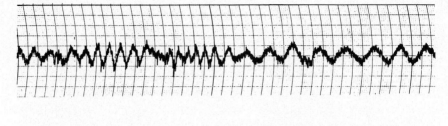

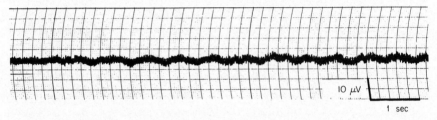

10 μV

1 sec

FIG. 3-7.   Comparison of induced voltages superimposed on the basic noise level by moving 2 parallel electrode wires toward and away from each other over a range of about 4 in. Two 30-gauge wire leads, 1 ft long, were connected to a dummy animal resistance of 15,000 Ω and were anchored at each end to prevent noise arising from motion at connection points. The bottom trace shows the attenuation achieved by having each wire shielded and grounded.

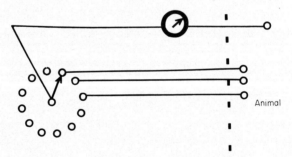

Animal

FIG. 3-8.   Simple circuit employing a rotary switch for rapid testing of interelectrode resistances.

V. Physiologic Artifacts

A. SKIN POTENTIALS

Cells of the skin generate slowly changing voltages. Also, autonomic control of sweat glands causes skin resistance to change, a phenomenon called the galvanic skin reflex (GSR); a decreased resistance occurs during emotional stress. If recording electrodes have a steady voltage difference between them, and most EEG electrodes do, slow inter-electrode resistance changes will cause slow voltage fluctuations in the EEG records. These artifacts can be minimized by selecting electrode pairs with little voltage difference between them. A more practical and more common approach is electronic filtering of such slow waves, using an amplifier time constant of about 0.3 sec (Chapter 5, Section III, B, 3).

B. ELECTROCARDIOGRAPHIC (EKG) SIGNALS

Potentials from the heart are very large, and under appropriate re-cording conditions can be recorded from any part of the body. The EKG voltages in the head region are large relative to the EEG, as can be demonstrated by recording between one electrode on the head and another on the neck. When both electrodes are on the head, the EKG signal is applied more or less equally to both amplifier inputs, and because differential amplifiers reject in-phase signals of equal magnitude (Chapter 4, Section I, D), the EKG does not appear in the EEG. There is one common situation where the EKG does appear in the EEG, and that is when one electrode of a pair has a significantly higher resistance than the other. This has the effect of impressing different EKG voltages on the amplifier grids, causing the EKG voltage difference to be ampli-fied (Fig. 3-9).

C. MUSCLE POTENTIALS

Potentials from the muscles of the head, especially temporal muscles of such species as dogs and cats, are common sources of artifact in the scalp-derived EEG. These potentials are spikelike and of high frequency and incidence. In a conscious animal, these potentials can be quite severe unless the animal is lying quietly without any face or jaw movements. Even when dogs or cats are in surgical planes of anesthesia, muscle potentials may appear in one or more leads (Figs. 3-9 and 3-10). For this reason, the author's own opinion is that anesthesia, or some other drug-induced restraint, is imperative for routine clinical EEG studies in dogs and cats (Klemm and Mallo, 1966; refer to Chapter 7).

Temporal muscle potential artifact presents much less of a problem in other animal species, such as rats and rabbits, which have relatively less muscle mass. In all species, the artifacts can be avoided by implant-ing electrodes in the skull and insulating them with dental cement from adjacent muscle and connective tissue. However, this surgical solution, although common in basic research, is usually not feasible for routine clinical EEGs.

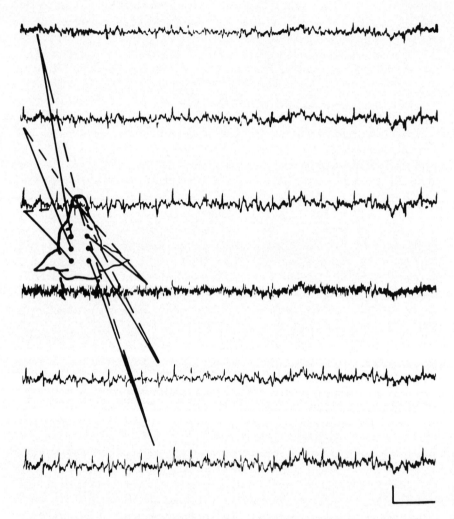

Fig. 3-9.   Illustration of electrocardiographic artifact appearing in all leads. The record illustrates higher amplitude of the artifact in the more posterior leads, indicating that potentials are greater there. However, differential amplifier characteristics could account for amplitude differences. Even if electrocardiographic potentials were equally distributed, the connection scheme used would result in greater amplification of occipital potentials. Traces also reveal muscle potential artifacts in the right frontal region, even though the dog was in a surgical plane of anesthesia. Calibrations: 20 μV; 1 sec.

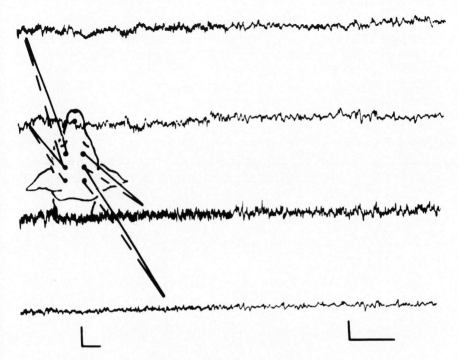

Fig. 3-10.   Illustration of muscle potential artifacts (right frontal–central region) in an anesthetized dog. Records are shown at 2 paper speeds. Calibrations: 20 μV; 1 sec.

D. THE EEG ITSELF

The EEG is a good example of the philosophy that "One man's noise is another man's signal." As mentioned in Chapter 1, the EEG contains activity ranging from DC to around a thousand waves per second (with intracerebral electrodes). Most investigators are only interested in the usual EEG frequency range of 1–50 waves/sec, and thus they consider anything else as noise. The researcher studying DC or multiple unit activity might consider conventional EEG frequencies as noise.

For practical reasons, which are discussed elsewhere, it is usually not advisable to record the entire brain spectrum of activity simultaneously on the same channel. If one wishes to examine the entire spectrum, it is best to do it in stages or to record simultaneously with separate channels. For example, assuming the use of nonpolarizable electrodes and appropriate electronic filters, the investigator would separately record DC activity, a conventional EEG, and an oscilloscope trace of fast waves and unit activity.

The conventional EEG also can be considered as noise if one is studying evoked potentials that may be present in, but masked by, the background EEG. Digital computer averaging techniques (Chapter 5, Section III, B, 5) are commonly used to reduce the amplitude of background EEG activity while simultaneously increasing the amplitude of small evoked responses.

VI. Motion Artifacts

Motion in the electrode region, of whatever origin, causes potentials to be generated at the electrode–tissue interface. Although certain electrode designs can reduce such artifacts (Chapter 2, Section II, A), they still may be quite prominent.

A. RESPIRATION

Respiratory movements are often reflected in the skin of the head and cause EEG electrodes to move with respect to the skin and thus cause artifacts. The artifacts are usually irregular slow waves of large voltage (Fig. 3-11). The best way to detect the presence of such artifacts is to mark on the EEG record each time a breath is taking place. If these marks coincide with large voltage EEG waves, one should strongly suspect them as artifact.

B. BALLISTOCARDIOGRAPHIC MOTION

These artifacts—rhythmic, large, slow waves—are caused by pulsations in blood vessels (Fig. 3-12). Such interference may occur anytime electrodes overlie large pulsating vessels; moving the electrode slightly often solves the problem. The artifacts also can be quite prominent when a reference electrode (Chapter 5, Section I, B) is placed on an ear that vibrates with blood pulsations.

C. EYE MOVEMENTS

Particularly in scalp recordings, artifacts often arise from blinking of eyelids or movements of the eyes. These artifacts usually take the form of isolated large voltage waves; the magnitude varies with species and with electrode placement. Ocular movement artifacts in chickens (Paulson, 1964) are illustrated in Fig. 3-13.

Ocular potential artifacts recently have been incriminated in contributing to the "alpha" rhythm of human EEGs (Lippold and Novotny,

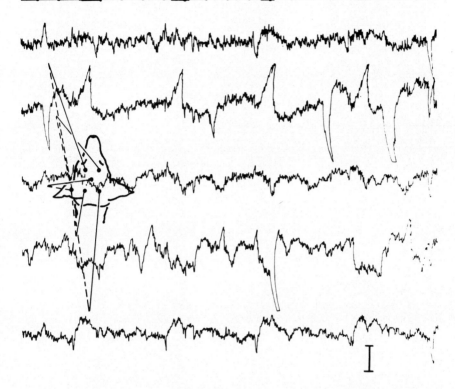

Fig. 3-11. Respiratory artifacts of high voltage, long duration, taken from an anesthetized dog. The artifacts are identified by their coincidence with breathing movements (indicated by the downward deflection marks on the time-mark line). Calibrations: 50 μV; 1 sec.

1968). These authors propose that the alpha rhythm actually results from an interaction between corneo-retinal potential and tremors of extraocular muscles. To support the contention, they bathed the closed eyes of humans with water of various temperatures; cold water slowed tremors and decreased the alpha frequency, whereas hot water had opposite effects. Control bathing of other parts of the face had no such effects. If this hypothesis can be confirmed, it means that many EEGs over the years have been misinterpreted.

Artifacts are especially prominent when DC recording amplifiers are used. The study by Wurtz (1965) revealed that mechanical movements of the eyeballs produced shifts in so-called "ultraslow" potentials of the brain (Fig. 3-14). These shifts had no consistent polarity; the magnitude of shift was less with transcortical recording than with recording against a frontal sinus reference electrode. Other movements of the unre-

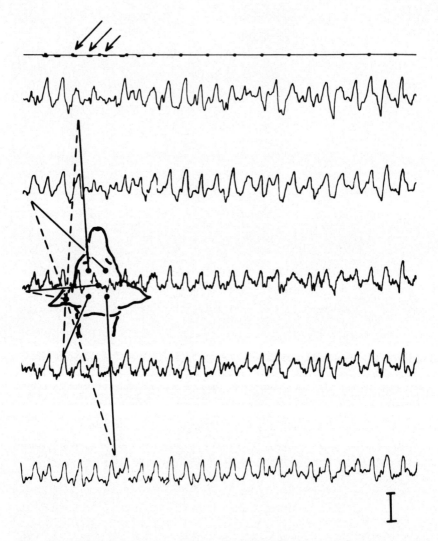

FIG. 3-12. Ballistocardiographic artifacts of regular high voltage, long duration, taken from an anesthetized dog. The artifacts are synchronized with the heartbeat, some of which are identified by arrows at the downward deflection along the time-mark line. Calibrations: 50 μV; 1 sec.

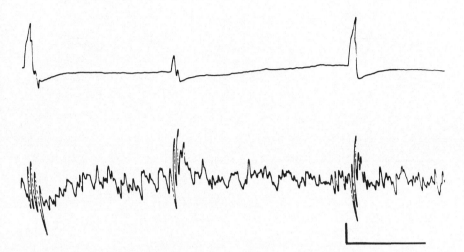

Fig. 3-13. Artifacts in scalp EEG (lower trace) originating from ocular movements (upper trace) of an unrestrained chicken. Calibrations: 50 μV; 1 sec. (Courtesy Dr. D. Coulter, Iowa State University.)

strained cat that produced ultraslow potential shifts were limited mainly to head shaking (Fig. 3-15).

D. General Movements

Most any type of body movement will cause motion artifacts, due to relative motion between lead wires as well as to electrode motion. The waveform of such artifacts is quite variable (Fig. 3-16) and is sometimes impossible to avoid (Fig. 3-17).

Other unusual potentials are generated during such acts as chewing and lip smacking (Fig. 6-15). It is difficult to say whether these are artifact potentials or are neural potentials being generated in the circuits that control such motor acts.

If experimental conditions require movement, as in behavioral studies, the best solution is to use fixed electrodes (Chapter 2, Section II, B), immovable connector contacts, and shielded, low-noise cables. Animals should be observed closely so that artifacts in the record can be identified.

The problem of cable movement in unrestrained animals creates not only electric noise but also causes twisting and kinking of cable, resulting in cable deterioration and restriction of movement. Slip-ring electric

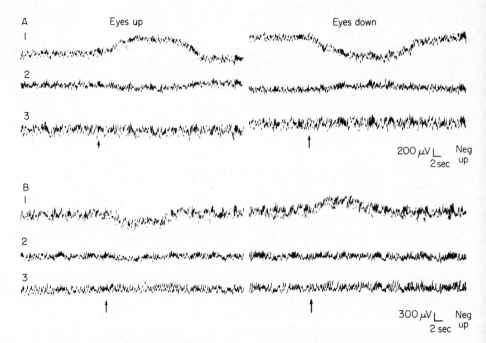

Fig. 3-14. Ultraslow potential shifts arising from mechanically produced movement of the eyes in the anesthetized cat. Arrows indicate initiation of movement. In A, recordings are between middle suprasylvian gyrus and frontal bone (1), occipital bone (2), and subcortical white matter (3). In B, recording is transcortical: sigmoid gyri (1), middle suprasylvian gyri (2), and posterior lateral gyri (3). (Wurtz, 1965.)

connectors are availabe to minimize this problem,[7] but they do introduce electric noise during turning. Noise can be reduced by use of mercury-filled cable couplers, such as the one devised by Sutton and Miller (1963).[8] Wires in the recording cable are connected to wires mounted on free-moving ball bearings. As the animal and cable turn, the wires rotate freely in mercury-filled grooves that are electrically connected to the recorder. No attenuation or distortion of the signal appears on records obtained through this coupler. Artifacts are still possible, however, and the magnitude is proportional to interelectrode resistance. Figure 3-18 illustrates the artifacts produced by gentle

[7]Available from Lehigh Valley Electronics, Inc., Fogelsville, Pennsylvania.
[8]Available from Laboratory Concepts, Inc., Bronx, New York; Lehigh Valley Electronics, Fogelsville, Pennsylvania. (The connector supplied with this unit is too noisy; it should be replaced with a locking connector. Better yet, the cable leads should be soldered directly to the wires that turn in the mercury.)

twirling of a low-noise cable (Microdot) connected at one end to a resistor and to a mercury cable coupler at the other end. Mundl (1967) suggests that these potentials result mainly from mercury's vibration against the statically charged plastic lining the grooves. He advocates the use of paper insulation between mercury-filled metal grooves and the use of platinum wire in the mercury pools.

One of the best ways to avoid cable artifacts is to use telemetry, which is such an expensive alternative that it often is not feasible. Telemetry also permits unrestricted movements, which is especially important in studies of EEG correlates of natural behavior. A full discussion of tele-

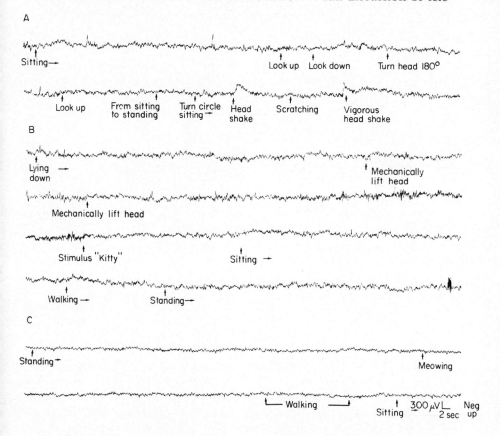

Fig. 3-15. Effect of movement and posture on ultraslow potentials of cortex. Recording is transcortical from sigmoid gyri. The records within A, B, and C are continuous; each line is 1¾ min long. Records A and B are from the pre-enucleated animal; record C is from the same animal after bilateral enucleation of the eyes. Pulling on the lead cord produced the mechanical lifting of the cat's head. In the last line of B, the cat walked to the window of the observation cage and looked out into the laboratory. (Wurtz, 1965.)

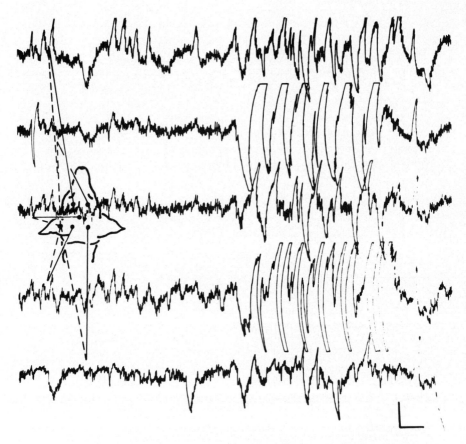

Fig. 3-16. General movement artifacts recorded from an unanesthetized dog. The artifacts are characterized by irregularity, high voltage, and long duration. All leads also exhibit lower voltage, faster activity due to muscle potentials. Calibrations: 50 μV; 1 sec.

metry is beyond the scope of this book (refer to Caceres, 1965; Ko and Neuman, 1967; MacKay, 1968). Suffice it to say that EEG telemetry requires a great deal of sophisticated instrumentation. The simultaneous telemetry of multiple data channels requires multiplexing circuitry and a high degree of miniaturization of transmitter components.

A four-channel device about the size of a cigarette pack has been developed by Hambrecht (1963). There also are several EEG telemetry transmitters on the market.[9] The Medtronics' unit, for example, con-

[9] A complete survey of commercially available units and their specifications is found in BIAC publication M12, available from the American Institute of Biological Sciences, Washington, D.C.

tains 8 channels, is smaller than a cigarette pack, has a range of 100 ft, and costs about $4500. Future developments in electronic ultraminiaturization should eventually improve transmitter performance and lower the cost.

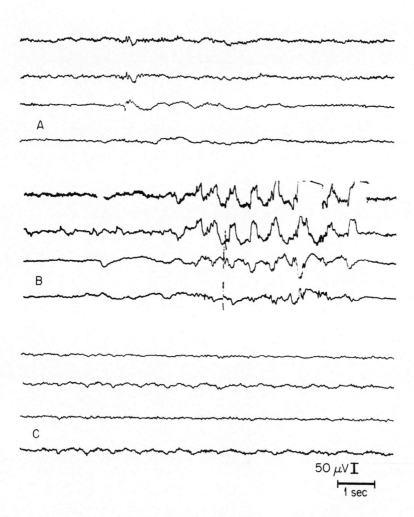

Fig. 3-17. Artifacts produced by subtle movements in unanesthetized dogs. A: Mixture of fast and slow wave artifacts produced by eyelid blinks followed by eyeball movements; B: high voltage artifacts produced by licking, chewing, and swallowing movements; C: rhythmic, 1/sec waves in second and fourth traces due to panting. (Redding, 1965.)

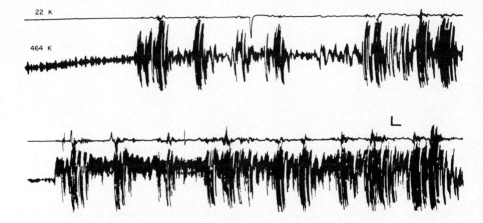

Fig. 3-18.   Artifacts generated by twirling a low-noise cable that connected at the animal end with resistors [22,000 (22 K) and 464,000 (464 K) Ω] and at the recorder end by means of a bearing that turned cable contacts in a mercury pool. Upper pair of traces show recordings obtained when the cable shield was grounded: lower pair reveal recordings with an ungrounded shield. Calibrations: 50 μV; 1 sec.

REFERENCES

Bureš, J., Petráň, M., and Zachar, J., eds. (1967). "Electrophysiological Methods in Biological Research," 3rd rev. ed. Academic Press, New York.

Caceres, C. A., ed. (1965). "Biomedical Telemetry." Academic Press, New York.

Hambrecht, F. T. (1963). A multichannel electroencephalographic telemetering system. Tech. Rept. No. 413. Massachusetts Institute of Technology, Cambridge, Massachusetts.

Kamp, A., Kok, M. L., and DeQuartel, F. W. (1965). A multiwire cable for recording from moving subjects. *Electroencephalog. Clin. Neurophysiol.* 18, 422–423.

Kay, R. H. (1964). "Experimental Biology." Reinhold, New York.

Klemm, W. R. (1965). Technical aspects of electroencephalography in animal research. *Am. J. Vet. Res.* 26, 1237–1248.

Klemm, W. R., and Mallo, G. L. (1966). Clinical electroencephalography in anesthetized small animals. *J. Am. Vet. Med. Assoc.* 148, 1038–1042.

Ko, W. H., and Neuman, M. R. (1967). Implant biotelemetry and microelectronics. *Science* 156, 351–360.

Lee, B. (1967). A shielded sound-attenuating chamber. *Psychophysiology* 3, 255–257.

Lippold, O. C. J., and Novotny, G. E. K. (1968). Tremor of the extra-ocular muscles as the generator of alpha rhythm: Cooling of the orbit in man. *J. Physiol. (London)* 194, 28P.

MacKay, R. S. (1968). "Bio-medical Telemetry." Wiley, New York.

Mundl, W. J. (1967). An improved swivel for recording from behaving subjects. *Electroencephalog. Clin. Neurophysiol.* 23, 483–485.

Nastuk, W. L., ed. (1964). "Physical Techniques in Biological Research," Vol. 5. Academic Press, New York.

Paulson, G. (1964). The avian EEG: An artifact associated with ocular movement. *Electroencephalog. Clin. Neurophysiol.* 16, 611–613.

Smullin, L. D., and Haus, H. A., eds. (1959). "Noise in Electron Devices." Wiley, New York.

Stacy, R. W. (1960). "Essentials of Biological and Medical Electronics." McGraw-Hill, New York.

Sutton, D., and Miller, J. M. (1963). Implanted electrodes: Cable coupler for elimination of movement artifact. *Science* **140**, 988–989.

Thompson, N. P., and Yarbrough, R. B. (1967). The shielding of electroencephalographic laboratories. *Psychophysiology* **4**, 244–248.

Whitfield, I. C. (1959). "An Introduction to Electronics for Physiological Workers." Macmillan, New York.

Wurtz, R. H. (1965). Steady potential shifts during arousal and deep sleep in the cat. *Electroencephalog. Clin. Neurophysiol.* **18**, 649–662.

Yanof, H. M. (1965). "Biomedical Electronics." F. Davis, Philadelphia, Pennsylvania.

4

Electronic Recording Systems

I. Electronic Principles of Special Relevance

A. CATHODE (EMITTER) FOLLOWERS

A special electronic circuit, called a cathode follower (or emitter follower in transistor circuits), is commonly used to raise the input impedance of amplifiers without simultaneously increasing capacitance relative to input resistance. The circuitry is interposed between the electrodes and the first amplifier stage, positioned close to the biologic preparation to reduce cable capacity.

High amplifier input impedance is especially needed when interelectrode impedance is high, as it always is with microelectrodes and sometimes is with implanted gross electrodes. The ratio of amplifier input impedance to interelectrode impedance determines how much of the biologic signal is passed on for amplification (Fig. 4-1A).

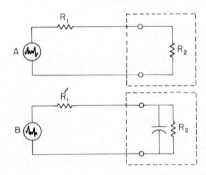

FIG. 4-1.   A: Illustration of how bioelectric voltages are distributed across interelectrode resistance (R_1) and the amplifier input resistance (R_2), which are in series. B: Illustration of how input capacitance can shunt high-frequency current away from the input resistance.

The figure illustrates a recording condition involving electrodes with high impedance (R_1). With electrodes coupled to amplifier input, current flow in this circuit develops voltages across both resistors; the total of these individual voltages must equal the applied voltage from the tissue. If in Fig. 4-1A we assume an interelectrode resistance of 1 megohm and an amplifier input impedance of 1 megohm, the voltage generated by tissue is divided equally across the 2 resistances. In other words, only ½ of the bioelectric signal is actually available for further amplification. This could be compensated for by added amplifying elements. However, the initial low signal-to-noise ratio could never be compensated, because subsequent amplification would amplify signal and noise equally. For this reason, amplifier inputs should have a high ratio of input impedance to interelectrode impedance.

Another associated source of signal distortion is the capacitance, which is always present across amplifier inputs; this comes from air gaps and cable insulation and is electrically equivalent to a capacitor in parallel with the amplifier input resistance (Fig. 4-1B). Even if the resistance values chosen, such as 1 and 10 megohms, are more favorable than in Fig. 4-1A, a problem is created by the capacitor's ability to shunt high-frequency current away from the input resistance. When the bioelectric signal contains high-frequency components, as with action potentials, the capacitor will likely offer less resistance to flow than the resistor, thus diverting a portion of the current away from the input resistance. The voltage developed across the resistance will thus be reduced, and the observed waveform will be a distorted version of the real one.

Cathode followers not only provide high input impedance but also reduce capacitative shunting of high frequencies because the cathode potential follows the grid potential by nearly the same amount. The extent of shunting can be determined by observing the distortion of known square waves that have been applied through the system.

The basic principles of cathode-follower function can be explained from Fig. 4-3 if we assume that the output resistor is placed in the cathode arm of the circuit instead of the plate arm. As a positive signal, for example, is impressed upon the grid, more current flows through the tube and through the cathode, developing voltage across the cathode resistor that is then coupled to a conventional amplifier. The cathode resistor is also coupled to the input, and voltage is fed back into the input. The cathode voltage "follows" the input voltage, producing no gain but preserving the phase characteristics of the input signal.

More detailed theory is provided by Kay (1964) and Suprynowicz (1966). Construction details are provided by Bureš *et al.* (1967), who also discuss balanced, or differential, cathode followers.

B. NEGATIVE CAPACITANCE ELECTROMETERS

Recording signals from microelectrodes imposes many demands on the quality of instrumentation. One of the more important requirements is for very high input impedance. Because electrode impedance is so high, amplifier input impedance must be great enough to prevent excessive loss of signal (refer to Section I, A). Another problem with microelectrode recording is the inevitable capacitance associated with the amplifier input and connecting cables. A capacitance as small as 20 pF shunts high-frequency components of the signal to ground, and rise time of square wave is degraded to about 400 μsec. If that capacitance were reduced to 1 pF, there would be a 20-fold improvement in rise time. Fortunately, the so-called negative capacitance electrometer has been developed recently[1] that partially neutralizes input capacity. Neutralization is achieved by applying an in-phase feedback from the output of a fixed-gain amplifier to the grid of the input tube through a properly chosen capacitor. The important specifications include a slow rate of drift (less than 1 mV/hr); low grid current (about 10^{-10}A) to prevent polarization of the cell under study; high input impedance (about 10^{12} Ω) to prevent signal loss; a high degree of capacitance neutralization ability (about 100 pF); and a low noise level at high source impedance.

Microelectrode recording requires a decision on whether electrodes should be placed extra- or intracellularly. Extracellular recording provides only a partial and somewhat distorted picture of neuronal activity. However, for many purposes extracellular methods are quite satisfactory. In addition, there are some advantages not found with intracellular methods: More cells can be sampled in a given time and simultaneous sampling of several cells is possible (refer also to comments on multiple unit recording in Chapter 5, Section III, B, 3). Identification of action potentials that are generated by different cells is usually based on differences in amplitude. Although action potentials of the same amplitude may come from the same or different neurons, potentials of differing amplitude must come from different neurons (unless neuronal-electrode distance changes).

Intracellular recording, when DC amplifiers are used, does offer a considerable advantage in that MP levels can be assessed. Also, MP

---

[1]Block Engineering, Cambridge, Massachusetts; Grass Instrument Company, Quincy, Massachusetts; Keithley Instruments, Cleveland, Ohio; Electronics for Life Sciences, Rockville, Maryland; Bioelectric Instruments, Hastings-on-Hudson, New York.

oscillations and their relations to action potentials and the EEG can be studied (Chapter 1).

C. AMPLIFIERS

The small magnitude of brain electric activity requires amplification to the point where signals can be observed on an oscilloscope or pen writer. Before discussing how this amplification can be achieved, it is first necessary to introduce concepts of how amplification, or *gain*, are quantified.

Gain can refer to increases in voltage, current, or power (current times voltage). Emphasis in electrobiology is given to voltage, which is easier to measure than current. Power is also important because it is necessary to activate the galvanometer coils in a pen recorder.

Engineers prefer thinking in terms of electric power. They have developed a logarithmic scheme for quantifying changes in power, either increase or decrease, based on the unit called the *decibel*. The decibel (db) is defined as

$$db = 10 \log P_2/P_1$$

where P_1 = initial power value and P_2 = the changed power value.

EEG traces, which are actually plots of voltage as a function of time, do not indicate electric power. Power cannot even be correctly calculated. Impedance, and consequently current flow, varies in different regions of the brain; even in a given region, impedance probably changes with changes in function of the neuronal pool in that region.

Thus, EEGs are usually quantified in terms of voltage. Some EEG manufacturers state their specifications in terms of voltage. For example, a frequency filter setting may be described as that setting at which a given frequency is attenuated to ½ the actual amplitude, that is, the amplitude without filtration.

However, the electronic industry as a whole uses the decibel system. Since biologists are not used to thinking logarithmically, and since the important EEG parameter is voltage, we sometimes need a means of converting decibels to percentage voltage change.

Decibels can be redefined in terms of voltage, rather than in terms of power. Since power equals voltage times current ($P = EI$) and since current equals voltage divided by impedance ($I = E/Z$), then power can be restated as $P = E^2/Z$. Note that this assumes a stable impedance, which is reasonable for instruments but not for living tissue.

Decibels can thus be redefined as

$$db = 10 \log \frac{E_2{}^2/Z_2}{E_1{}^2/Z_1} \quad = 10 \log \frac{E_2{}^2}{E_1{}^2} \quad = 20 \log \frac{E_2}{E_1}$$

For various decibel values, the pecentage change in voltage can be calculated using the above formulas; Fig. 4-2 is a plot of the percentage–decibel relation.

The simplest type of amplifying device is the *triode*. It consists of 3 main elements enclosed in a glass-sealed vacuum: (1) a *cathode*, which when heated and connected to an electron source emits electrons; (2) a *plate*, which when made positive collects the emitted electrons; and (3) a *grid*, interposed between cathode and plate, which regulates electron flow from cathode to plate by the bioelectric signal it receives.

Placement of a triode in an amplifying circuit is illustrated in Fig. 4-3. The left-hand battery serves to *bias* the grid, i.e., put a charge on it, which in this case tends to restrict electron flow from the cathode by the

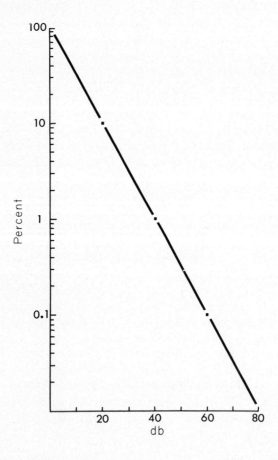

FIG. 4-2.   Percentage change in voltage as a function of decibel values (db).

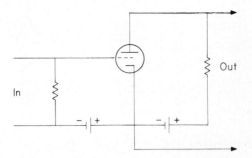

FIG. 4-3. A simple triode amplifier circuit.

mutual repulsive forces of electrons. An input signal at the grid will change the degree of this biasing and, consequently, change the amount of current flowing from the right-hand battery to the plate and back to the battery. A negative input signal will make the grid more negative, decreasing electron flow from cathode to plate; conversely, a positive input signal will make the grid less negative, increasing electron flow from cathode to plate. As current flows through the tube, output voltage develops across the load resistor of the output portion of the circuit. This voltage is exactly out of phase with the input signal. To illustrate, a positive grid voltage increases electron flow through the tube and load resistor; this makes the top of the resistor negative with respect to the bottom.

How does amplification occur? The close spatial relations between grid and cathode enable small changes in grid voltage to have great effects on current flow. These large changes in current flow cause large voltage changes at the load resistor. Thus, the output voltage is amplified, i.e., it is larger than the voltage change occurring at the grid.

Transistors are being used increasingly in amplifiers. They have several important advantages over vacuum tubes, such as smaller size, more shock resistance, and lower power requirements. Disadvantages include excessive noise (a problem that is being solved) and, commonly, feedback from the output.

Manufacturers incorporate transistors into their equipment to various degrees, ranging from partially transistorized circuitry (Grass) to completely transistorized circuitry (Beckman).

Transistor functions are thoroughly reviewed elsewhere (Kiver, 1960; Kosow, 1962; Bureš *et al.*, 1967). For our purposes we can say that transistors consist of pieces of semiconductor material sandwiched together. The 2 types of material, positive (P type) and electron-rich (N type), are created by adding a few atoms of an impurity (arsenic-

excess electrons; boron, gallium, or indium-excess positivity) to a semi-conductor crystal such as germanium.

When a P–N junction is formed by putting P and N crystals together, one would expect the charge difference to neutralize, as electrons distribute in the P crystal. This does not happen, however, because the P crystal is only slightly positive, and it contains many negative atoms that repel incoming electrons. Current (i.e., electrons) will flow, however, if the repelling forces are neutralized by applying voltage of proper polarity across the P–N junction; this is the so-called "forward bias" condition.

A properly biased P–N junction (diode) can serve as a rectifier, allowing current flow in only one direction. It cannot, by itself, be used for amplification.

Amplification is possible by joining 3 pieces of crystal, either P–N–P or N–P–N, with suitable connecting leads and biasing. The N–P–N type will be used to explain how amplification occurs (Fig. 4-4). The P crystal in the circuit is represented by the vertical line within the circle, and it is called the "base." The base connects with 2 N crystals, which are represented by the angular lines; the arrow shows the direction of *positive* current flow from N to P to N. The line with the arrow is called the "emitter" (because it emits electrons), and the other line is called the "collector" (because it collects electrons from the emitter). In other words, electrons flow in the direction opposite to the arrow direction.

Note that the base of P crystal is connected to an input. There is a similarity here to the input grid of a vacuum tube, in that signal applied to the grid (base) regulates current flow from the cathode (emitter) to the plate (collector).

The circuit illustrated is analogous to the tube circuit discussed previously in that the emitter (cathode) is common to both input and output portions of the circuit. This arrangement is thus called "common-emitter" (or common-cathode).

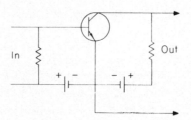

Fig. 4-4. A simple amplifier circuit involving an N–P–N transistor. For a P–N–P transistor, the battery polarities would be reversed.

The battery arrangement tends to promote current flow through the transistor. Electrons emerge from both batteries and flow together in the emitter lead. Upon entering the emitter-base junction, about 5% of the electrons flow through the base to the positive pole of the left-hand current. Why do not *all* of the electrons flow in this direction?

The fact is that most electrons would go through the base of P crystal if the crystal were large. It is intentionally made very small so that most electrons are impelled completely through the base into the collector, whereupon the electrons "see" the positive attractive force of the right-hand battery.

Where does amplification come from? The answer lies in the fact that small changes in base polarity cause large changes in collector current. Recall that 95% of current through a transistor flows through the emitter–collector circuit, developing voltage across the load resistor at the output. The rate at which electrons flow through the emitter–collector junction is controlled by the bias voltage on the base; a positive signal would aid emitter–collector flow, and a negative signal would restrict it. Small changes in base bias cause large changes in emitter–collector current. Because base current is very small, a change in emitter–base bias will have a far greater effect on emitter–collector current than on base current. The voltage developed across the output resistor is thus amplified.

The analogy here to common-cathode vacuum tube operation is quite striking. In a tube, recall that the electrons leaving the cathode (i.e., the emitter) are governed by the grid voltage. Most of the electrons leaving the cathode enter the plate (i.e., the collector). Of course, one can go too far in making analogies between transistors and vacuum tubes.

Tubes and transistors can be connected in 2 other ways: common-grid (common-base) and common-plate (common-collector). The connection scheme used depends on the desired input–output impedances, input–output phase relations, voltage gain, and power gain. In EEG amplifiers, the amplifying elements are usually cascaded in series to achieve the high gains necessary. The initial amplification is accomplished in preamplifiers, which usually have a gain of about 1000. The amplified voltage is then fed into power amplifiers that build up current levels sufficiently to activate pen-writing elements.

In recent years a special type of amplifier has been introduced called the *operational amplifier*. Theoretical discussions of the circuitry are beyond the scope of this book (see Swinnen, 1968); several manufacturers (Philbrick, Nexus *et al.*) have excellent manuals. Operational amplifiers are quite versatile and can be designed with an infinite input impedance, making them valuable in measuring voltage from high impedance sources. The amplifiers also can be designed for extremely high gain. Other uses include precision current monitoring, electronic integration, and follower circuits. Operational amplifiers are even useful when arranged for differential voltage amplification, a subject discussed next.

D. DIFFERENTIAL AMPLIFICATION

Brain electric activity is recorded with so-called "differential amplifiers," also known as "push–pull amplifiers." There are 2 main reasons for using this type of amplifier: (1) it avoids interaction between channels when simultaneously recording from several electrode pairs and (2) it selectively rejects 60 Hz interference.

The circuit is so constructed that it *amplifies only signals that differ from each other at the 2 inputs.* As a result, one electrode could be connected to several amplifier channels without causing interaction, whereas connecting an electrode to several cathodes of conventional amplifiers would cause the voltage at that electrode to influence current flow in all channels. Also, if differential inputs receive 60 Hz activity of equal voltage, the interference will not be recorded at all. In practice, this discrimination against 60 Hz is relative, because the interference at each input is seldom exactly of the same voltage.

Differential amplifiers are usually only used for the first stages of amplification, with the amplified bioelectric signal passed on in sequence through a series of conventional amplifier stages. This scheme is basically similar to that found in many oscilloscopes and pen recorders.

A simplified differential circuit is illustrated in Fig. 4-5. Before discussing how this circuit functions, it may be useful to review how amplification occurs if the amplifier is not operated differentially (many oscilloscopes have switches that make differential operation optional). With the switches in the A position, amplification would be nondifferential. Consider, for example, the case where 2 electrodes connect an animal to the X input and ground. Suppose that a positive pulse were generated under the animal electrode which connects to the X input. In the case of the X input, this pulse would cause G_1 to become positive with respect to ground. The positive charge at G_1 would increase the flow of electrons from the cathode to the anode in tube 1. As electrons flowed through R_1, a voltage would develop that would be passed on to the next stage for further amplification.

Now let us consider the case when switches are turned to points AB. Again, a positive signal applied to the X input would develop a voltage at G_1, which would be amplified. What if the animal had generated positive charges at both places on his head where the electrodes were

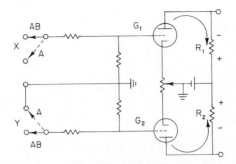

Fig. 4-5. Simplified circuit to illustrate the principles of differential amplification (when signal is applied to X and Y inputs and with switches in AB position). Direction of *electron* flow through the tubes is indicated when positive signal is applied simultaneously to both grids (G_1 and G_2).

connected and these pulses were in phase and of equal magnitude? One must now consider what happens at the Y input and at G_2. At the same time that G_1 becomes positive with respect to ground, the positive charge at Y causes G_2 to develop a positive charge with respect to ground. The positive G_2 accelerates electrons through tube 2, and a consequent voltage develops across R_2 that is the same magnitude but of opposite polarity, as that produced across R_1 by electron flow through tube 1. Thus, no net potential is impressed upon subsequent amplification stages, and there would be no amplification of the original signals applied to X and Y inputs.

However, amplification would occur in the case where the 2 inputs are charged by signals that differ in any way (voltage, frequency, or phase). Consider, for example, the situation where 2 identical spikes are simultaneously generated that have the same voltage but opposite polarity, that is, they are 180° out of phase. Suppose the one at X were negative; this would restrict current flow through tube 1 and prevent development of a load voltage across R_1. The positive spike at Y would cause a positive charge on G_2 and thus develop a load voltage across R_2 that would be passed on to the next stage for further amplification.

E. Galvanometer Principles

Most EEG writer systems involve movement of a coil in which current is flowing. The current in the coil represents the amplified EEG signal; this current's interaction with a surrounding magnetic field rotates the coil proportionately to the amount and polarity of current.

As current flows in the coil, the coil moves; movement will be restricted by tension that develops on a spring on the torsion wire suspension of the coil. As the angle of the coil's turn increases, so does the restraining force of the torsion spring. At a certain angle of deflection, the spring's force equals the electromagnetic force causing the rotation, and the pen remains in that position as long as the signal does not change.

A pen suspended on the rotating coil subscribes an arc. Such recordings are called curvilinear and are subject to a certain amount of amplitude distortion from the lack of true vertical deflection. This curving is especially prominent with wider pen excursions. EEG traces of 1–2 cm excursion are not distorted much; but many types of recording, such as blood pressure, respiration, force, etc., may require wide pen excursions. Under such circumstances, amplitude cannot be measured directly with a ruler but must be measured along the curved path. Correlation of sample points along the curve with time and correlation of simultaneous phase relations in several channels can be difficult; for this reason, many manufacturers provide specially ruled paper for curvilinear recordings.

Several manufacturers supply rectilinear write-out for their recorders that avoids the problems just mentioned. Rectilinear recording is achieved by employing a mechanical correction linkage or servo system for the coil galvanometer. Rectilinear write-out devices usually have a poorer high-frequency response than curvilinear systems, mainly because rectilinear coupling is mechanically complicated.

Moving-coil galvanometers have practical limits, based mainly on inertia and momentum. For example, if a signal is suddenly applied to the coil in a resting position, inertia will cause some lag in response, a factor that limits fidelity of high-frequency recording. There is also a lag tendency due to friction of the pen or paper. Finally, momentum of a rapidly moving body tends to cause overshoot of the equilibrium deflection position. Correction of these problems makes galvanometer design quite an art, in spite of the apparently simple principles involved.

Commercial recorders usually have properly adjusted galvanometers. However, it is often useful periodically to adjust pen pressure, until one obtains the fastest rise time without overshoot.

High-frequency limitations of galvanometers are usually the limiting factors on a recorder's performance. In this respect, no EEG machine is any better than its galvanometers. Calibration of a galvanometer's frequency response is easily achieved by applying sine-wave signals of increasing frequency. At some point the amplitude of those sine waves will progressively decrease. The upper limit of faithfully reproducing high frequencies is about 150 Hz in the best moving-coil pen writers.

Although a good pen galvanometer is easily adequate for EEG frequencies, other write-out devices are more suitable for higher frequencies because they have less mass, inertia, and momentum. One device employs a d'Arsonval movement that deflects a light beam instead of turning a pen; this is the so-called mirror galvanometer. Mirrors can be made very small, and the whole coil can be quite delicate. The light beam is ultimately deflected onto light-sensitive paper. With ultraviolet light and special paper, no photographic developing is needed. The low inertia of such systems[2] permits faithful reproduction of frequencies of 2000 Hz or more.

The most conspicuous advantages of such systems, in addition to better high-frequency response, is near rectilinear traces (due to long beam length), absence of pen-clogging problems, and adjustable line width. The obvious disadvantage is expense, due to the photographic recording paper needed. The paper also should be stored in darkness.

F. Oscilloscope Monitoring

In many ways the oscilloscope is the most versatile instrument in the bioelectric laboratory. Its special attribute is the ability to reproduce fast transients, although it can be used to display any electric signal, biologic or otherwise.

The basic principles of oscilloscope operation are illustrated in Fig. 4-6. A heated cathode emits free electrons that are accelerated toward a fluorescent screen target by high voltage. The beam can be vertically positioned at any level on the screen, and it sweeps from left to right, followed by an essentially instantaneous flyback and restart of another sweep. Built-in adjustments permit changing the sweep rate to either very fast or very slow; this provides an adjustable horizontal time base.

The term "time base" derives from the fact that most modern scopes have sweep speeds calibrated in terms of a direct unit of time for a given distance of spot travel across the screen. The units of distance, usually centimeters and fractions thereof, are marked on transparent plastic that covers the tube face. Although it is common practice to think and speak of time bases in terms of relative sweep speeds (horizontal velocity of the spot), measurement of waveform durations is easiest when using the reciprocal of speed: time per division (such as milliseconds per centimeter).

Some investigations require fast sweeps and others slow sweeps, and

[2]Sanborn Division, Hewlett Packard Company, Waltham, Massachusetts; Honeywell Company, Denver, Colorado; Varian Company, Palo Alto, California.

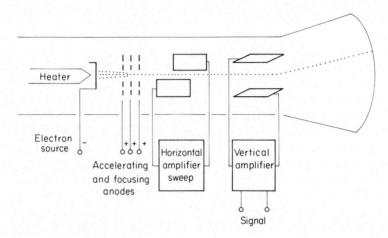

Fɪɢ. 4-6. Simplified diagram, illustrating the major features of a cathode-ray oscilloscope.

a versatile scope should be capable of both. Appropriate time–base settings depend on the phenomena being studied. For example, individual action potentials of nerve are best observed with a total sweep time of about 5 msec. Whatever the total range of sweep speeds may be, continuous coverage is usually available, along with discrete calibrated steps controlled by switches.

Sweep linearity is an important factor that is seldom specified by manufacturers. There are various forms of nonlinearity. To check for accuracy and linearity, it is common practice to observe a sine-wave signal of known frequency.

Sometimes it is desirable to display parts of waveforms that occur considerably later than do suitable sweep triggering signals. Such waveforms always can be displayed on sweeps that last long enough, but if the duration is short compared to the length of the sweep, an accurate examination may not be possible. The need to expand (magnify) the display for the time interval during which a particular event occurs is apparent. Portions of sweeps may be magnified by increasing the gain of the horizontal amplifier (allowing either or both ends of the sweep to go off-screen) and positioning the display so that the desired portion is on-screen. This is a simple way to meet the need. Another way is to generate suitably delayed sweep triggering signals so that fast sweeps may be triggered just prior to the moments when the signal to be examined occurs.

Although not commonly used in electrobiology as an *x-y* plotter, some oscilloscopes have horizontal axis and vertical axis amplifiers. Thus, one can apply signals to horizontal deflection plates that bend the beam proportional to an input voltage or one can use the *x* axis as a preset, linear sweep speed.

Displaying pulses of short duration and low repetition frequency is quite difficult unless the pulses themselves drive or trigger the sweeps. Commonly, a sweep can be started by an internal triggering pulse that is fired whenever a preset voltage is reached by the bioelectric signal. Such practice accommodates almost any type of signal, except those that have very high frequency.

Triggering level controls are available that permit selection of the voltage level at which a signal will trigger a sweep. The controls provide selection of either positive or negative voltages, so that triggering can be set to occur only with a given polarity.

Triggering controls offer an additional important feature, that of "ranging" or "phasing." Triggering can be delayed deliberately for long periods while a slowly changing triggering signal is climbing or falling to the selected triggering level. The display of a sine wave, for example, may be displaced horizontally by triggering at different levels on either of its 2 slopes.

Normally, bioelectric voltages deflect the sweeping electron beam either up or down, depending on polarity. Deflection is accomplished by applying the amplified signal to deflection plates that when charged either repel or attract electrons, thus causing bending of the beam.

The faithfulness with which a deflection system displays fast-rising step signals (square waves) is termed its transient response. The most common response distortions are overshoot, ringing, and reflections from impedance discontinuities in the vertical signal delay line. These forms of distortion will cause step signals to have spikes, squiggles, or bumps when they actually do not.

The major qualification generally sought in a scope is adequate "rise time" or adequate high-frequency sine-wave response. Rise time is the more important specification for faster scopes, and passband (bandwidth) is the more frequently used specification for slower scopes. The two will be closely related mathematically, however, when fast step signals produce little or no overshoot or ringing. The product of rise time and frequency response should produce a factor whose value lies between 0.33 and 0.35 when transient response is optimum. Factors larger than 0.35 probably indicate overshoot in excess of 2%, while those larger than 0.4 probably indicate overshoot in excess of 5%.

Sensitivity, like frequency response and rise time, is one of the prime factors determining the suitability of a scope for a particular application. When the utmost in sensitivity is required, some bandwidth must be sacrificed to reduce electric noise.

Most modern oscilloscopes have DC-coupled deflection systems, which are essential for displaying undistorted low-frequency signals. Usually, AC coupling is also made available, primarily to block DC input voltages that might otherwise drive the whole display off the screen.

High-gain, DC-coupled amplifiers are apt to drift appreciably. Long warm-up periods are sometimes required to reduce this drift. The maximum drift is often specified in terms of millivolts per hour. The degree of position change of course will depend on the deflection factor selected. For instance, if the factor is 1 mV/cm and the drift specification is 1 mV/hr, the drift in a 1-hr period should not be greater than 1 cm. Generally, drift per hour is of little consequence, because measurements are usually taken for only a few seconds or minutes.

Many scopes have differential amplifier circuits (Section I, D) that reject, to a high degree, any signals that are equal in amplitude and phase at both inputs. The degree to which unwanted signals can be rejected is termed "common-mode rejection ratio." A rejection ratio of 100:1 indicates that the amplitude of the displayed common-mode signal is only 1% of what might be displayed without differential input. Significant rejection of common-mode signals much larger in amplitude than the signal to be displayed requires very high rejection ratios of several thousand to 1. Most differential amplifiers do not maintain maximum rejection ratios for weeks at a time, but adjustments usually allow reestablishment of maximum rejection.

A very useful type of dual-input amplifier is one that can pass either of two input signals one at a time to permit viewing either signal without disturbing connections. Comparison of the 2 signals thus is possible. Manual switching, available on some scopes, is the simplest method, but electronic switching permits simultaneous viewing of 2 signals. Since the 2 signals trace out separate displays, scopes with built-in electronic switches are commonly called "dual-trace" scopes (some have 8 or more traces). They should not be confused with "dual-beam" scopes that have 2 entirely separate vertical deflection systems and sometimes even independent time–base controls. Dual-beam scopes therefore are much more versatile, but they are also more expensive.

The major disadvantage of oscilloscopes is the problem in obtaining a permanent record of the beam deflections. This is usually achieved photographically, a relatively expensive and time-consuming method. Cameras used can range from very elaborate motion-picture cameras[3]

---

[3]Such cameras are available from Grass Instrument Company, Quincy, Massachusetts and Lehigh Valley Electronics, Fogelsville, Pennsylvania.

to simple, single-lens, reflex 35-mm cameras. With the latter the shutter is held open while the beam sweeps. Close-up lenses and a lightproof camera mount are essential.[4]

Another solution to the reproduction problem is the use of digital, storage oscilloscopes. Digitization provides other advantages as well, but cost may be prohibitive. Another, less expensive, solution is offered by "variable persistence" scopes (Hewlett–Packard) in which the beam image can be retained for more than 1 min.

A partial solution is available with a newly developed interface device[5] that is installed between any standard scope and any standard x-y plotter. The interface unit samples a *repetitive* waveform many times in order to obtain a tracing. In this process only the waveform repeats itself, and asynchronous noise does not appreciably affect the tracing. Unfortunately, such a system could not be used to record EEGs or other aperiodic potentials; it could be used to advantage for recording evoked responses. The resultant thin-line pen plot is a substantial enlargement of the scope trace, making detailed analysis easier.

A final problem associated with reproducing scope displays is that fast-rising waveforms, such as action potentials, are often poorly illuminated. The fading of the beam during rapid deflections is difficult to view, either directly or after reproduction. A special vertical beam intensifier has been developed that solves this problem.[6] The problem is also said to be alleviated with use of variable persistence scopes.

II. Electroencephalographs

A. SPECIFICATIONS AND COMMERCIALLY AVAILABLE RECORDERS

On the following pages a few of the many types of EEG machines are illustrated. Decisions as to preference for a given model and manufacturer must be based on individual need and financial resources. It therefore is suggested that the buyer obtain descriptive brochures and price lists from each manufacturer and make direct comparisons. Table 4-1 lists some of the leading suppliers of EEG recorders.

Each user will have his own set of specification priorities. However, the remainder of this chapter will discuss the features one could reasonably expect to find in a quality recorder. In general, these specifications should be considered as minimum.

---

[4]More detailed photographic instructions are available from Kodak Job Sheet No. 1, Eastman Kodak Company, Rochester, New York.

[5]Model 1001, Pacific Measurements, Inc., Palo Alto, California.

[6]Medical Instruments, Inc., Portland, Oregon.

TABLE 4-1
COMPANIES MAKING ELECTROENCEPHALOGRAPHS

Ahrend-van Gogh	Distributed by Technical Equipment Marketing Associates, Crawley, Sussex, England
Alvar	Montreuil, France
Brush Division, Clevite Company	Cleveland, Ohio
Cambridge	Ossining, New York
Electro-Medical Engineering	Burbank, California
Elema-Schonander	Stockholm-Solna, Sweden
Grass	Quincy, Massachusetts
Kogyo (Lehigh Valley Electronics)	Fogelsville, Pennsylvania
Lexington	Waltham, Massachusetts
Minneapolis-Honeywell	Denver, Colorado
Sanborn Division, Hewlett Packard	Waltham, Massachusetts
Spinco Division, Beckman	Palo Alto, California
Schwarzer	Framingham, Massachusetts

EEG recorders should have flexible filter settings, both for high and low frequencies. High-frequency filters are useful for eliminating noise from the traces (noise increases with increasing bandwidth). Care must be taken not to filter out meaningful signal, as high-frequency filtration produces conspicuous distortion (Fig. 4-7). Recorders also should be equipped with specific 60-Hz filters for use under temporarily poor recording conditions. However, 60-Hz filters distort other frequencies to an extent (Chapter 5, Section III, B, 3) and use is discouraged. There is no substitute for properly shielded and grounded preparations (Chapter 3, Section IV).

Low-frequency filtration settings also are very important. Conventionally, filtration settings are expressed in terms of "time constant," which in the case of slow frequencies refers to the time required for a pulse to fall two-thirds of the way toward the base line. The influences of various time constants and their relation to ½-amplitude values is illustrated (Fig. 4-8). Typical time constants for recording various bioelectric phenomena include at least 500 msec for electrocardiograms, 10–30 msec for electromyograms, and 100 msec for electroencephalograms. Choice of a low-frequency cut-off point should not be made arbitrarily but in reference to specific recording conditions. This is conveniently determined by simultaneous recording of the same signal with different time constants. The shortest time constant that does not

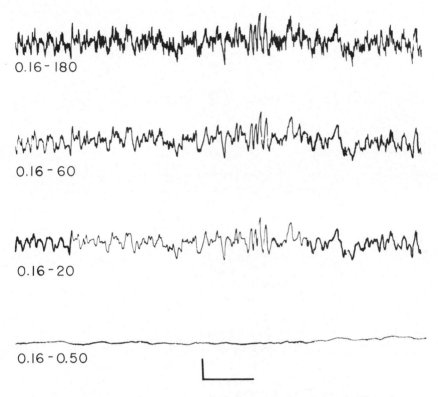

0.16 - 180

0.16 - 60

0.16 - 20

0.16 - 0.50

FIG. 4-7. High-frequency filtration effects on the EEG, illustrating the distortion produced by simultaneous recording of a signal with varying cut-off frequencies, at which the
signal is attenuated to 70% of maximum amplitude. Calibrations: 20 μV; 1 sec.

distort the slowest components of the trace should be selected (Fig. 4-9).
Use of unnecessarily long time constants increases the chance of recording motion artifacts that often are of low frequency. Distortion of EEG
traces by using excessively fast time constants is illustrated in Fig. 4-10.

EEG recorders should be equipped with electrode switching capability
so that connection schemes can be altered easily without repositioning
electrodes. Such switching operations require an electrode plug-in
board, which in turn is connected to selector switches. Switches should
be wired so that a given electrode can be connected to either G_1 or G_2
inputs of the preamplifier.[7] Most commercial recorders provide such

[7] By physiologic convention, most EEG instruments are wired so that a negative signal
at G_1 causes an upward pen deflection; engineering convention is the opposite — negative
signals deflect downward.

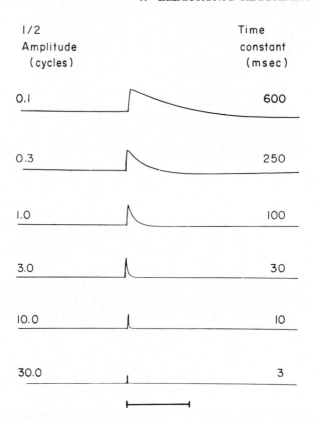

FIG. 4-8.   Effect of low-frequency filtration on a 50 μV DC calibration signal supplied simultaneously to all channels. Filtration settings are expressed in terms of ½-amplitude frequency and its equivalent in time-constant values. Note not only the difference in fall times but also the lower peak amplitudes that occur with faster time constants. Calibration: 1 sec.

switches, some of them being quite elaborate. Switching devices also can be made using rotary switches and shielded cable. It is useful to include electrode resistance test jacks in the circuitry (refer also to Chapter 2, Section I, A).

Variable paper speed controls are essential. Although the conventional paper speed is 30 mm/sec, other speeds are often useful. For example, 60 mm/sec is useful for more detailed inspection of high frequencies, especially 60-Hz noise. The slower speed of 15 mm/sec is useful for long, continuous recording sessions; the overall activity can be monitored without excessive use of paper. Even slower speeds are

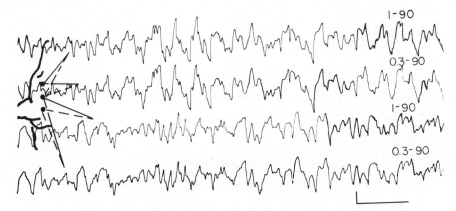

Fig. 4-9. Simultaneous recording of EEG from deeply anesthetized dog with ½-amplitude low-frequency cut-off points of 0.3 and 1 Hz. Identical nature of traces of same signal indicate that in this case a cut-off point of 1 is desirable. Calibrations: 20 μV; 1 sec. (Klemm, 1968.)

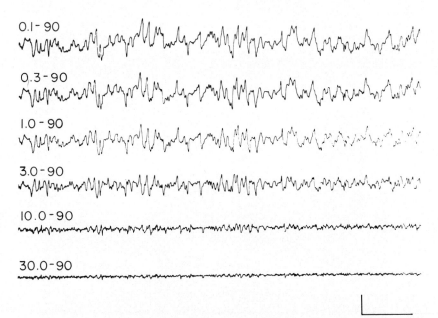

Fig. 4.10. Effect of low-frequency filtration upon the EEG. The same signal from an anesthetized dog was recorded simultaneously with the indicated ½-amplitude frequency cut-off points. The ½-amplitude frequency setting was 90 Hz in each instance. Calibrations: 20 μV; 1 sec.

sometimes used when conspicuous paroxysmal activity is to be observed over a long period. Slow recording speeds are also valuable for long-term monitoring of desynchronized and synchronized patterns, as in sleep studies.

Most manufacturers supply paper[8] for their machines (Figs. 4-11– 4-16). Paper is expensive, but this is because a quality, smooth surface

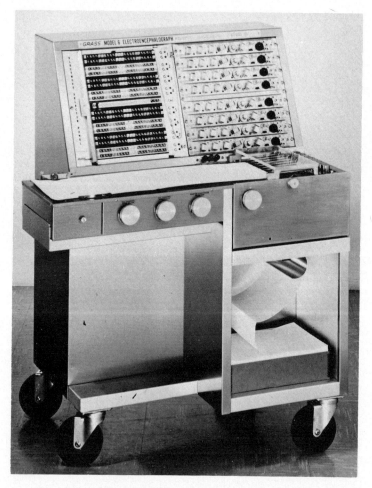

Fig. 4-11.   Grass Model 6 recorder (Grass Instrument Company).

[8]Paper of various sizes for most commercial recorders can be obtained from Graphic Controls Company, Buffalo, New York.

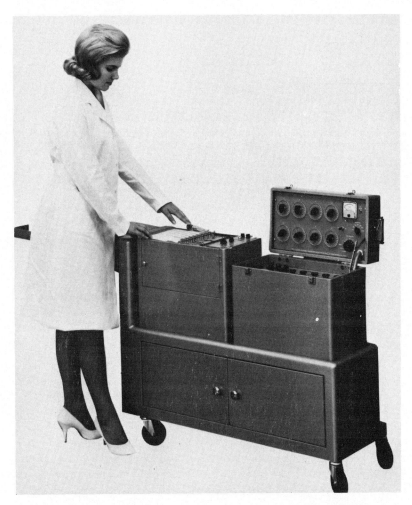

Fig. 4-12. Beckman Model T portable recorder (Spinco Division, Beckman Instruments Company).

paper is needed to reduce pen friction, which improves frequency response and prolongs pen life.

Amplifier specifications are particularly important. Input impedance should be at least 1 megohm. The common-mode rejection ratio should be 1:2000 or better. Noise level, with 10,000 Ω across the input and a bandwidth of 1–90 Hz (½-amplitude) should be less than 4 μV. Gain settings should be variable, with a maximum sensitivity of 2 μV/mm. In addition, each channel should have a gain equalizer control, which is

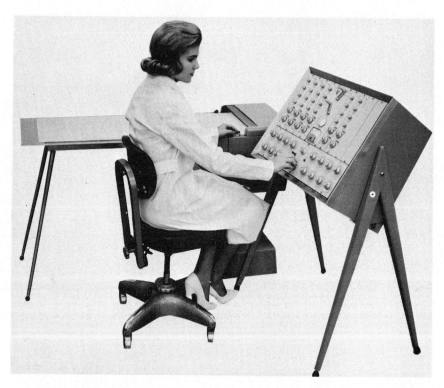

FIG. 4-13. Beckman Model TC recorder (Spinco Division, Beckman Instruments Company).

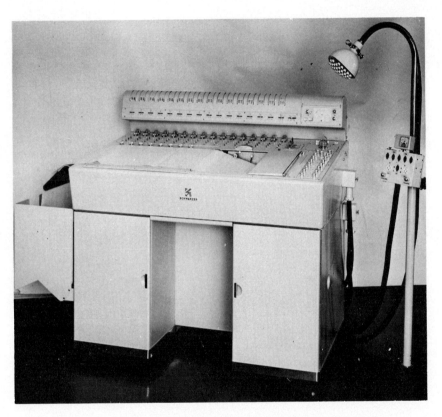

Fɪɢ. 4-14.   Schwarzer Model EPS 16 recorder (Schwarzer Company).

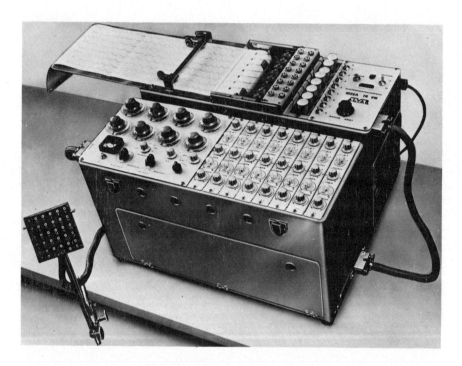

Fɪɢ. 4-15.   Alvar Reega VIII portable recorder (Alvar Electronic Company).

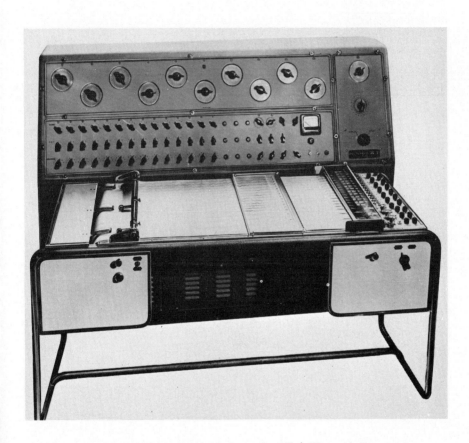

FIG. 4-16.   Alvar Reega XX channel recorder (Alvar Electronic Company).

a fine adjustment permitting all amplifiers to have exactly the same gain. Amplifiers should have deblocking circuits that hasten the recovery time from transient overloads caused by artifact signals.

Built-in calibration voltages are important. They are especially convenient when arranged so that all channels can be calibrated simultaneously.

Output monitor jacks are essential for oscilloscope monitoring or computer analyses. The signal condition at the output jack should meet IRIG standards.

Finally, a time and event marker should be available.

REFERENCES

Bureš, J., Petráň, M., and Zachar, J., eds. (1967). "Electrophysiological Methods in Biological Research," 3rd rev. ed. Academic Press, New York.

Kay, R. H. (1964). "Experimental Biology." Reinhold, New York.

Kiver, M. S. (1960). "Understanding Transistors." Allied Radio, Chicago, Illinois.

Klemm, W. R. (1968). Subjective and quantitative analyses of the electroencephalogram of anesthetized normal dogs: Control data for clinical diagnosis. *Am. J. Vet. Res.* **29**, 1267–1277.

Kosow, I. L. (1962). "Transistors." Prentice-Hall, Englewood Cliffs, New Jersey.

Suprynowicz, V. A. (1966). "Introduction to Electronics for Students of Biology, Chemistry, and Medicine." Addison-Wesley, Reading, Massachusetts.

Swinnen, M. E. T. (1968). The design of biomedical instrumentation made easy through the use of operational amplifiers. *Psychophysiol.* **5**, 178–187.

5

Interpretation and Analysis of the EEG

I. Electrode Configurations

A. BIPOLAR

All EEGs are derived from bipolar (Mowery and Bennett, 1961) electrode arrangements, that is, a pair of electrodes. The term "monopolar" misleadingly implies recording from one electrode; in reality it refers to use of one of the electrodes on a reference area, such as an ear or the nose, which is relatively inactive electrically.

Both bipolar and reference recording contribute somewhat different information, due largely to the EEG amplifier's method of amplifying only *difference* of potential between the 2 electrodes. With bipolar recording, brain potentials at both electrodes are often relatively similar. If the *same* potential should appear simultaneously at both electrodes, no amplification would result, erroneously indicating absence of the potential. More commonly, various degrees of subtraction occur. For example, 2 simultaneously occurring potentials of the same shape and duration but of slightly different amplitude would be amplified to the extent that their amplitudes differed. Two simultaneously occurring potentials that were identical except for being 180° out of phase would be doubly amplified. These concepts are clearer with an understanding of differential amplification (Chapter 4, Section I, D).

Subtraction effects of bipolar recording account for the generally lower amplitude of bipolar recordings, as opposed to recordings with an inactive reference electrode (Figs. 5-5–5-8). How much subtraction and

127

consequent reduction of amplitude occurs with bipolar recording depends in large measure on the interelectrode distance. Widely separated electrodes are more likely to overlie areas of differing electric activity, thus registering greater potential difference between electrodes and resulting in higher voltages in the recorded EEG. Conversely, closely spaced electrodes often overlie potential fields that are similar at both electrodes, and thus less amplification occurs.

Clearly, the bipolar method produces a distorted and somewhat difficult-to-interpret EEG. One could reasonably question the value of such an approach, as some leading electroencephalographers have. However, there are a few advantages to bipolar recording that are sufficient to justify its use. Among these are the relative ease of distinguishing true brain potential from artifact, which normally does not occur in all channels as often as it does in reference recording. Another advantage is that localization of pathologic foci sometimes can be established with more certainty (Chapter 7). The advantages should become more apparent from further reading of this book.

B. Recording with a Reference Electrode (Monopolar)

Such recording refers to registration of the potential difference between one "active" electrode on the head or in the brain and another "inactive" electrode placed over an area that is relatively less active electrically. The "inactive" reference electrode is always connected to the G_2 amplifier grid (refer to Chapter 4, Section I, D), so that a negative discharge at the active electrode causes the recording pen to deflect upward. Cancellation effects are not as prominent as with bipolar methods and, as a consequence, EEG voltages are larger (Figs. 5-6–5-8). Activity that appears in a given channel can be interpreted as originating near the "active" electrode of the pair. Activity that appears simultaneously in several leads originates nearest the electrode in which such activity is most conspicuous.

The limitation of reference recording methods is that there is no perfectly suitable reference point for the inactive electrode. The animal body is an electric volume conductor, albeit complex, in which potentials are widely distributed from many sources. The ear or bridge of the nose is often selected for the reference electrode and, although brain potentials are small in these regions, they are nonetheless present (Fig. 5-1). There are, of course, more inactive regions on the body (with respect to brain potentials), but recording from regions further away from the head often introduces electrocardiographic or muscle potentials.

Another disadvantage of reference recording is that an artifact poten-

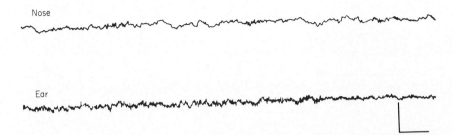

Fig. 5-1. Activity present at 2 commonly chosen reference electrode sites, as recorded from bipolar electrodes 5 cm apart on a lightly anesthetized dog. The high frequencies in the trace from the ear probably are muscle potentials, although at that time no such potentials were present in bipolar leads recording from directly over the temporal skull region. Calibration marks: 20 μV; 1 sec. (Klemm, 1968a.)

tial at the reference electrode will cause the artifact to appear in all recording channels. When recording bizarre activity, it may be difficult to establish whether such activity is artifact or genuine brain potential. This problem can be illustrated by the studies of electrographic seizures during animal "hypnosis" in which a nasal reference electrode was used (Klemm, 1966). The proof that these potentials were not artifact was established by bipolar recordings and by simultaneous recording over areas that could most likely be contributing artifact (Fig. 5-2).

Several modifications of the reference technique are used in human clinical electroencephalography, all of which are aimed at reducing the effect of activity at the reference electrode. One such technique involves the use of 2 reference electrodes, one located on the neck and another on the chest, which have a potentiometer between them for balancing out electrocardiographic potentials. Another common technique is the use of the so-called "average reference electrode" (reviewed by Barthel, 1961). The basic concept is to connect all the electrodes together through equal parallel resistances of 0.5–2 megohms to serve as a reference electrode. The total resistance of such an average electrode is equal to R/n, where R is the value of one resistor and n is the number of resistors used. The parallel resistances act as voltage dividers, reducing the voltage at any one electrode n times for n number of electrodes. Thus, in the Goldman system used in human electroencephalography, 10–16 scalp electrodes are brought together at the G_2 input to serve as the reference. Such an averaging system works quite well, except when there is large, synchronous, and diffuse activity common to all electrodes making up the reference. Better results could be obtained if the average electrodes were placed on relatively inactive regions such as the nose.

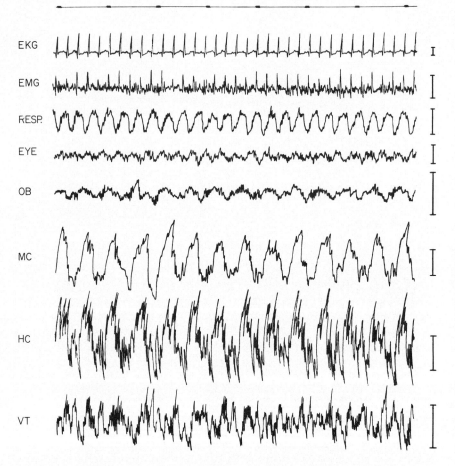

EKG

EMG

RESP.

EYE

OB

MC

HC

VT

FIG. 5-2.   Electrographic seizures obtained with nasal reference recording. Bipolar records illustrate the improbability that the seizure activity in the 3 bottom traces is due to artifact. Recordings from the most likely sources of artifact (potentials from the heart, muscle, respiratory movements, and olfactory bulb) are shown during a dyclonine-induced seizure in a "hypnotized" rabbit. EKG, electrocardiogram; EMG, nuchal electromyogram; RESP., respiration movement potentials; EYE, eye movement potentials; OB, olfactory bulb; MC, motor cortex; HC, hippocampus; VT, ventral thalamus. Calibrations: 50 μV and 1 sec (top line of illustration). (Klemm, 1966.)

The lower voltages at the nose should cancel toward zero more readily than the higher voltages on the cranium proper. Also, widespread synchronous activity still could be detected because the voltage would be much less at the nose. There are practical difficulties, however, in the inconvenience of attaching extra electrodes to a small region.

C. STANDARDIZED ELECTRODE ARRANGEMENTS

For reproducibility, comparative purposes, or detection of focal abnormalities, scalp electrodes need to be placed in standardized positions. Ideally, electrode positions should be measured from skull landmarks. There should be adequate coverage of all parts of the head, and electrodes should cover homologous regions on the two sides of the head. In human clinical electroencephalography, many years elapsed before agreement could be reached on a standard electrode arrangement. In 1957 the so-called 10–20 system was approved (Jasper, 1958). The 10–20 referred to the percentage of the total circumferential length from the nasion to the inion (Fig. 5-3). Although most electroencephalographers accept and use this system, the difficulty in achieving unanimity is illustrated by several leading workers who criticized the system as being more geometric than electroencephalographic (Gibbs and Gibbs, 1964; Pampiglione, 1956). The system, however, does not preclude the use of other electrode positions. One commonly used position is in the pharynx, the so-called nasopharyngeal electrode, which is used in man to detect lesions of the uncus, hippocampus, and deep portions of the temporal lobe (Mavor and Hellen, 1964).

In clinical electroencephalography of animals, there is no standard scalp electrode arrangement, although the author has proposed an 8-electrode system and numbering scheme for dogs (Klemm, 1968b; Figs. 5-4 A and B) that is not dissimilar to a 10-electrode system advocated for use in children (Kagawa, 1962).

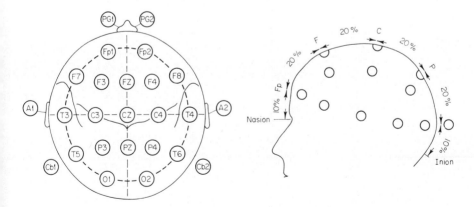

FIG. 5-3. Diagrams of a conventional electrode placement for clinical electroencephalography in humans. Drawing on the right illustrates the proportions used to determine interelectrode distances. (Redrawn from Jasper, 1958.)

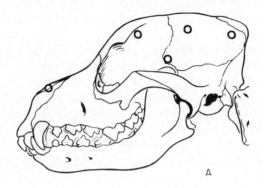

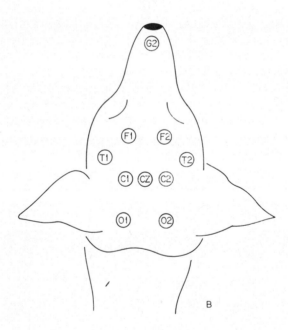

Fig. 5-4.   A: Suggested electrode position sites for scalp recording of electroencephalograms from the dog. Nasal electrode is used as a reference. (Klemm, 1968a.) B: Suggested electrode numbering scheme for clinical electroencephalography in dogs. (Klemm, 1968b.)

II. Frequency[1]-Amplitude-Phase Characteristics

A. BIPOLAR

Certain general rules of interpretation can be derived for bipolar recording. These rules apply equally to scalp or intracerebral recording and are derived from the fact that a differential amplifier discriminates against in-phase activity at its two grids and amplifies only *differing voltages*. Illustration of these principles can be found in the manuscript by Walter (1963).

A waveform that occurs in an area equally affecting two bipolar electrodes will not be amplified, because an equal charge is placed on the grids of the differential amplifier (Fig. 5-5).

Increasing distance between electrodes usually results in increased amplitude of recorded waveforms. Closely spaced electrodes are more likely to record from neuronal generators of similar activity, thereby resulting in more cancellation (Fig. 5-8).

A given wave will have the largest amplitude in the bipolar lead nearest the region where that wave originated, assuming each pair has the same interelectrode separation. The reason is that cancellation effects tend to occur in a fixed ratio in this instance and, at remote electrode pairs, can reduce the wave to imperceptibility.

A series of electrode pairs with fixed separation will record a waveform that originates far away with a low amplitude that is similar in each lead because of distance and cancellation effects.

Occurrence of a phase reversal of a given potential as a given bipolar pair is moved along a single path indicates that the waveform was generated at the point of phase inversion. This is due to the polarity arrangements of amplifier connections (see below). The technique is often used intracerebrally to identify signals from certain cell layers.

Many of these principles of interpretation are illustrated by the dog EEG, which contains several features that make it especially suitable, as will become apparent.

As illustrated in Fig. 5-6, bipolar recordings from linearly arranged scalp electrodes usually produce a great deal of out-of-phase activity between traces that originate from a common electrode. The reason for so much out-of-phase activity, often termed "phase inversion," is largely due to polarity of amplifier connections. For example, the row of 3 electrodes on the left side are so connected that electrode 2 influences the

---

[1]The term "frequency" is used in a special sense. Engineering usage usually refers to a repetitive waveform of uniform duration. Such repetitive waveforms do not occur in the EEG. Frequency of a given EEG wave refers to the number of waves that *would* occur in a second *if* that wave repeated itself continuously.

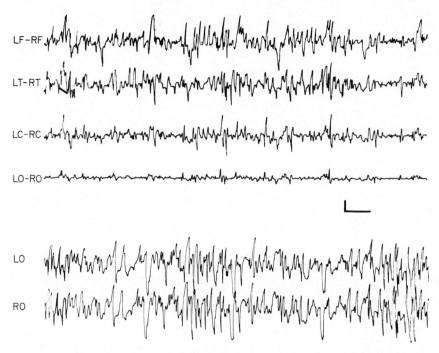

LF–RF

LT–RT

LC–RC

LO–RO

LO

RO

Fig. 5-5.   Illustration of voltage cancellation effects of differential recording. EEG was obtained from a 6-month-old cat, 2 months after an anesthetic accident in which the heart stopped and was eventually restarted. The top four traces are bipolar recordings; note especially the low voltage in the left occipital–right occipital (LO–RO) trace. This could misleadingly suggest that the occipital region was relatively inactive. On the contrary, recording each occipital electrode against a nasal reference revealed a great deal of activity. The almost exact duplication of waveforms from the two areas explains why there is little voltage difference to be amplified in a bipolar connection. Abbreviations represent left or right frontal (F), central (C), temporal (T), and occipital (O) electrode positions. Calibrations: 20 μV; 1 sec.

EEG in both channels 1 and 2. If a negative wave, for example, originated under electrode 2, it would be displayed upward in the channel 2 recording because the number 2 electrode is connected to G_1, which when negative deflects pens upward[2] (Chapter 4, Section I, D). That same negative wave, however, also influences channel 1 because electrode 2 is connected to it. Since in channel 1 the number 2 electrode is connected to G_2, the negativity will be displayed as a downward pen

[2]The following convention for amplifier polarity is generally accepted: The lead to an amplifier which, when made negative relative to the other lead, produces an upward deflection of the light beam or pen is referred to as "black" and in diagrams is drawn as a *solid* line. The other lead is referred to as "white" and is drawn as a *broken* line (Walter, 1963).

deflection—out of phase with the simultaneously occurring upward deflection in channel 2.

The electrode connections in the diagram are suggested for routine use because they permit localization of out-of-phase activity from a given hemisphere, longitudinally from the 3 linear electrodes and laterally from the fourth electrode.

This ability of bipolar arrangements to indicate the origin of individual waves is of major importance. If an abnormal EEG wave exists, indicating disease, bipolar methods can identify the origin and suggest the location of a brain lesion. Because out-of-phase activity is so conspicuous, even in normal animals, the initial key question involves a decision as to whether given out-of-phase waves are abnormal. Further discussion of this matter is found in Chapter 7.

Numerous bipolar arrangements are possible; one particularly useful arrangement is shown in Fig. 5-7. Contrary to the case where a given electrode is common to 2 channels, this transhemispheric arrangement produces a great deal of in-phase activity in normal animals. Except for amplitude, the traces appear almost identical, a reflection of relatively

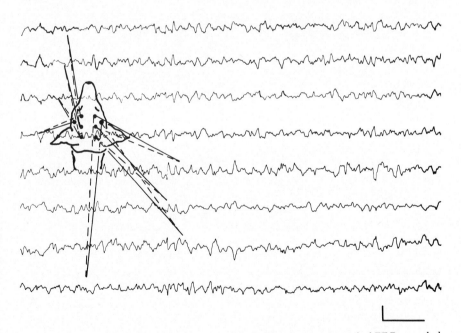

FIG. 5-6. Intrahemispheric bipolar recording arrangement and a typical EEG recorded during light anesthesia in a normal dog. Record indicates little amplitude difference between leads. Waveforms in each tracing are relatively dissimilar, with considerable out-of-phase activity. Calibrations: 20 μV; 1 sec. (Klemm, 1968a.)

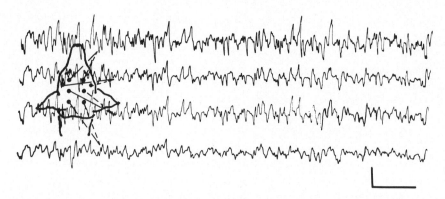

FIG. 5-7. Transhemispheric bipolar recording arrangement and a typical EEG recorded during light anesthesia in a normal dog. Record indicates a progressive decrease in amplitudes from anterior to posterior. Waveforms in each tracing are quite similar, and there is a great deal of in-phase activity. Amplitudes were larger than those from intrahemispheric bipolar records on this same animal. Calibrations: 20 μV; 1 sec. (Klemm, 1968a.)

uniform activity along the longitudinal axis of the cortex. Abnormal activity at any point along the cortical axis should be readily apparent by producing a conspicuous dissimilarity in one or more of the traces. The progressive anterior to posterior amplitude decrease may be due in part to signal attenuation by bone, which is quite thick over the occipital region of dogs. The smaller posterior potentials could be due to more transhemispheric synchrony of occipital cortex generators, thus resulting in more cancellation; however, reference recordings do not indicate any obvious anterior to posterior difference in transhemispheric symmetry. Amplitudes of transhemispheric EEGs tend to be larger than those of intrahemispheric records. This suggests less synchrony between transhemispheric cortical generators, resulting in greater interelectrode voltage difference and less voltage cancellation (see below).

B. RECORDS FROM REFERENCE RECORDING

Recording between active sites and a relatively inactive reference point produces still different EEG patterns (Fig. 5-8). One conspicuous difference is a higher amplitude than in bipolar recording. Because very little activity is present at a reference point, there is considerable difference in voltage between electrodes. Only differing voltages are amplified by differential amplifiers, and the trace amplitude therefore is large. In a bipolar arrangement, presence of significant activity at both electrodes, some of which has similar phase and amplitude, produces a degree of cancellation; there is less interelectrode voltage difference available for amplification. The progressive amplitude increase from anterior to posterior probably results from potential *difference* increase as "active" electrodes are further from the reference electrode. Occipital cortex could be generating larger potentials, but this seems unlikely because transhemispheric bipolar scalp recordings reveal lower amplitudes over occipital regions.

The records shown also illustrate similarity of waves originating from various electrodes over the same hemisphere. This suggests relatively uniform activity along the long axis of the cortex, as suggested previously by the bipolar recordings in Fig. 5-7. However, there is less similarity between hemispheres, suggesting a tendency for independent function and having great physiologic implications.

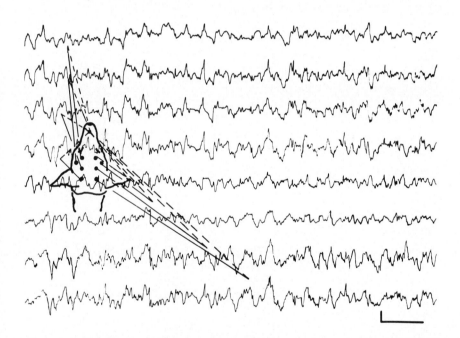

Fig. 5-8. Reference electrode recording arrangement and a typical EEG recorded during light anesthesia in a normal dog. Record indicates a progressive anterior-to-posterior increase in amplitude. Waveforms in each tracing from the same side are quite similar, and there is a great deal of in-phase activity; there is less similarity between hemispheres. Calibrations: 20 μV; 1 sec. (Klemm, 1968a.)

III. Data Analyses

Analysis techniques can be classified in 2 categories: those methods designed to evaluate what the eye sees and those that by certain mathematical and electronic operations quantify that which the eye does not see. In both categories there is increasing reliance on electronic devices, although visual analysis will always be a fundamental approach.

A. VISUAL OBSERVATIONS

The original technique for EEG analysis was the "eyeball" method, wherein records were visually scanned to identify important phase-amplitude-frequency characteristics of individual waves and wave patterns. Some examples of visual analysis were presented in the previous discussion on EEG interpretation. In spite of the computer revolution today, visual analysis is still the most common approach. Clearly such analysis has major disadvantages, such as the fallibility of human judgment and the impossibility of quantifying multiple channels of EEG data. On the other hand, automatic instrumental analysis methods have major disadvantages, too. For one, they have more limited "judgment" than humans; machines are rather "stupid" and can only rigidly perform analysis within the limits of their programs.[3] Moreover, instrumental analysis is usually accomplished for only one or a few facets of the total spectrum of EEG characteristics. Most instruments, even the most sophisticated, are programmed to analyze only certain specific features of an EEG, completely ignoring the others. The human brain can qualitatively evaluate all visible aspects of an EEG. No computer has yet matched the human ability to recognize patterns in the EEG.

For these reasons EEG analysis is not done by electronic means alone. In fact, many famous investigators steadfastly refuse to use any sort of automatic analysis, mainly because the *meaning* of the data is often unclear. Though this is the extreme position, it does illustrate a recognition of the limitations of instrumental analysis.

EEG data can be quantified visually, but this is very tedious. The tedium is reduced if one is only trying to describe unusual events within an EEG, such as spindles, seizures, or conspicuously slow or fast activity.

For measuring individual EEG wave durations and amplitudes, there are special ruler designs that simplify the process. The ruler devised by Sheatz (1964) is illustrated in full size in Fig. 5-9. The frequencies

---

[3]To really appreciate the problems of visual analysis or of programming a computer, the following exercise is recommended: Visually compute amplitude and wave-duration histograms from 10 sec of an EEG. In the process the magnitude of required judgment and arbitrary decisions should become abundantly clear. The problems are confounded further when using mathematical or electronic means to extract information that is not visible to the eye.

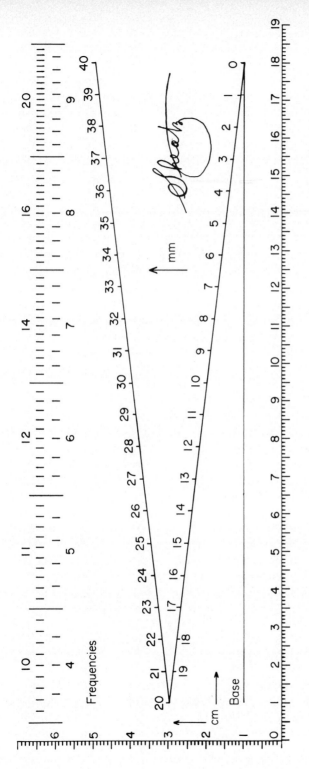

Fig. 5-9. EEG ruler. Left and lower lines calibrated in centimeters and millimeters. Ruler is reproduced here at its original size to permit contact prints. (Sheatz, 1964; U.S. Army photograph.)

numbered 4–20 are the cycles per second of any coinciding EEG rhythm at the standard paper speed of 30 mm/sec. Multiples or submultiples, of course, may be measured by estimation. For amplitude measurements, the lower solid line is moved along the lower limit of the amplitude to be measured until an inclined line touches the top of the amplitude; the vertical distance is read to the nearest numbered millimeter.

Other published ruler designs have been reported by Marshall (1955) and Turner (1955). A ruler that can be obtained by writing to the company is illustrated in full size in Fig. 5-10. All are designed for the standard paper speed, but multiples or submultiples can be estimated.

Paper speed and amplifier gain setting have a great influence on visual analysis. The usual paper speed of 30 mm/sec has been selected because at that speed most frequencies are sufficiently displayed for convenient and accurate estimation of their durations. However, this speed is not adequate for very fast frequencies (above about 40–50/sec). Slower paper speeds so compress each individual wave that accurate measurement is not possible. On the other hand, slow paper speeds can be useful if one wishes to scan long-time segments for pattern evaluation; a speed of 15 mm/sec is often a good compromise, permitting a reasonable estimate of individual wave durations as well as facilitating inspection of much data in a single eye span.

Amplifier gain setting must be taken into account during analysis, especially when comparing different EEGs. Comparison is made easier when the same gain is used for all EEG records. This is not always feasible, however, because in both scalp and intracerebral derivations, amplitudes may vary considerably among different animals and even among various regions within the same animal. The magnitude of amplification should be adjusted for clear observation of each individual wave. The gain should not be so high that the amplifiers are overloaded, which in a record appears as a chopped-off wave at the extreme excursion point of the pen. Gain should be high enough so that information contained in low voltage waves is not lost; there is some evidence that the usual gains employed in human electroencephalography may sometimes prevent detection of abnormal EEG waves (refer to Chapter 7).

B. Electronic Analyses

Such analyses involve processing of amplified EEGs with special electronic instruments. Most EEG recorders have special jacks for connecting the amplified signal to a tape recorder or special computing devices (IRIG standards should be met). More detail on instrumental

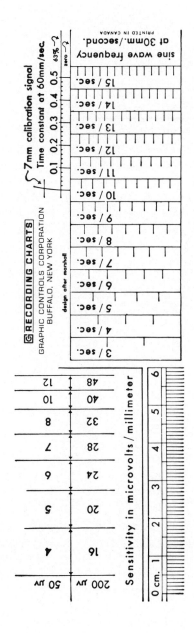

Fig. 5-10. Commercially available EEG ruler that can be obtained by writing the company. Ruler is reproduced at original size to permit contact prints. (Courtesy of Graphic Controls Corporation.)

analysis may be found in the books by Bures *et al.* (1967) and Rosenblith (1962).

Tape recorders are very useful for providing permanent storage of EEG data in a form that can readily be fed into computers. Their only serious disadvantage is that analyses are not performed "on-line," that is, during the actual experiment when adjustments of procedure may be necessary. Multichannel tape recorders with quality suitable for EEGs are expensive; some of the commercial sources are listed.[4]

Most electronic analysis modifies the original EEG. Moreover, many techniques reduce the data in that a continuous analog plot of voltage vs time is sampled at discrete points in time and converted to proportional, digital values that are subsequently computed in various ways (Maloney and Bradham, 1965; Ulam, 1964). Thus the advantages of objective quantification must be weighed against the disadvantages of arbitrary criteria and data reduction.

There are numerous electronic methods of analysis, many of which may evolve into more sophisticated and, hopefully, more meaningful techniques. The remainder of this chapter is devoted to a brief introduction to some of the methods. Each technique has its own advantages and limitations. There is no general agreement on which techniques are especially valuable, and for that reason detailed discussion of a given method is not presented. References to the literature cited should permit the reader to explore a given method in more detail.

1. Amplitude Analysis

One way to quantify the EEG is to measure amplitude of individual waves. This approach has been comprehensively reviewed recently (Goldstein and Beck, 1965).

One of the early techniques was to measure the amplitudes with a ruler and calculate averages or histograms. Electronic devices, so-called pulse-height analyzers, are now available that permit computation of amplitude histograms. These analyzers are based on the "window" principle, wherein a preset window is the threshold at which pulses or peaks of waves are counted. The number of pulses occurring at each threshold level can be tallied by electronic scalers.

Instrumentation for such devices is relatively simple and expense is not very prohibitive. The major disadvantage of such analysis is the emphasis placed on EEG amplitude; time relations are ignored. The

---

[4]Ampex Corporation, Redwood City, California; Electronic Design Laboratory, Philadelphia, Pennsylvania; Honeywell Electronic Medical Systems, Denver, Colorado; and Midwestern Instruments, Tulsa, Oklahoma.

importance of frequency content can be illustrated by a spike and a long duration wave with identical amplitudes; they obviously indicate quite different physiological states of the neuronal pools that generated them. EEG amplitude among various animals is affected by many variables that do not reflect brain function, such as surface area of electrodes, quality of electrode–tissue connection, variations in the extent of inter- posed insulating barriers like myelin, skull, and skin, and others. In the EEGs of symptom-free, and presumably normal dogs, for example, 2-fold differences in amplifier gain settings were often required to achieve equivalent pen excursions (Klemm, 1968a).

Amplitude analysis, however, can be important in relative evaluation on the same animal in which major changes in electrode–tissue im- pedance are unlikely.

2. Time and Interval Analysis

"Time" analysis is not a clear term, but it is sometimes used to mean a calculation of the number of EEG waves occurring in a given period of time. This can be done relatively easily by visual analysis. Electron- ically, it is done by circuitry that fires a pulse each time a voltage excur- sion occurs across a zero point (Ertl, 1965) or across a preselected discrimination threshold. Such devices can be constructed by using Schmitt trigger circuits (Bureš *et al.*, 1967). Also, most digital computers that sample an analog waveform can be programmed for such readout.

Interval histogram analysis, although more elegant, is based on the same principle of detecting excursions across zero or a discrimination level. The difference lies in the fact that the interval between excursion points is computed. This is most readily achieved by digital computers, which after sampling the analog waveform at various intervals convert the voltage sampled to proportional digital values. Once such conversion is accomplished, many computation modes are possible in addition to an interval histogram.

A major problem with time or interval histogram analysis is the arbitrary decisions required for filtration of the compounded EEG waveforms. As mentioned earlier, EEG waves in animals contain many small, high-frequency voltages that are superimposed upon larger and longer duration waves. Should these small components be computed? To do so would lessen sensitivity for detection of slow-wave phenom- ena. Omission of short-duration wave data presumes that such data are not important. These decisions are clearly not easy to make; they must be made in context with the experimental situation and with understanding gleaned from prior research. In the case of clinical

EEGs, for example, it is well established that disease is often indicated by a shift away from or toward the large, long duration waves (Chapter 7). Thus, removal of small, superimposed waves seems justified, and even desirable, because it increases the sensitivity for detection of shifts. A reasonable filtration setting would seem to be 1/2-amplitude at about 30 cps. A sample interval histogram from anesthetized normal dogs is shown in Fig. 5-11.

Another problem is the decision concerning sample size. What number of waves will provide a representative histogram? The answer will be dictated by the experimental situation and by how much variation occurs between successive 100-wave increments. In the case of the anesthetized normal dog, as few as 100 waves seems representative (Fig. 5-12), although perhaps more should be computed to increase reliability.

3. Spectral (Frequency) Analysis

EEGs can be analyzed in terms of their frequency content, a basically mathematical concept that is accomplished by computers. More than 100 years ago Fourier demonstrated that voltage–time functions could be described as the sum of trigometric (sine and cosine) series; for theoretical detail, consult Bureš et al. (1967). Such analysis is a very convenient way to analyze compounded waveforms such as the EEG (Chapter 1, Section III, A).

Fourier's approach allows one to look at a given compounded wave and calculate what settings on a series of sine-wave generators would permit a duplication of that waveform. In other words, the analysis tells what components are present in a compounded waveform.

The advantage of Fourier analysis should be obvious. The disadvantages, aside from the fact that some have questioned the appropriateness of Fourier analysis to the EEG (reviewed by Brazier, 1961), is the fact that information about transients and phase relations is lost in the computations.

As a practical matter, frequency content of EEGs is usually determined by a series of electronic filters. Electric filtration can facilitate analysis of the EEG because it separates the frequency components of the compounded EEG waves. Electric filters are basically designed to pass desired signals and reject undesired signals. "Band-pass" filters are used to pass a certain range of frequencies, filtering out all frequencies on the low and high sides of that band. The lower limit of this pass band is often referred to as the low-cutoff frequency and the upper limit as the high-cutoff frequency. Low-pass filters are used to preserve low fre-

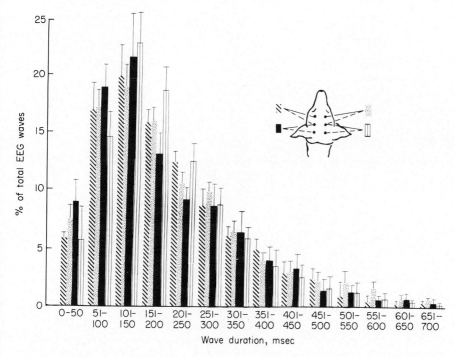

FIG. 5-11. Interval histogram averaged from intrahemispheric bipolar recordings of 7 normal dogs during deep barbiturate anesthesia. Deviations shown equal 1 SE. (Klemm, 1968a.)

quencies and filter out high frequencies, which is useful for recording ultraslow potentials of brain. Conversely, high-pass filters preserve high frequencies and filter out the low ones, which is useful for recording multiple action potentials from implanted electrodes.

The simplest type of filter is called "passive," and it contains only resistance, inductance, and capacitance.[5] Such filters are inexpensive and very reliable for frequencies above 200 cps. The source should be low impedance and should have considerable power, meaning that EEGs must be amplified before filtering.

A filter can be made by simply using resistance and capacitance, with the reactance of the capacity determining the frequencies that will be filtered (Suckling, 1961). For example, a 1-μF capacitor has a reactance of 16 Ω for 10,000 cps, 166 Ω for 1000 cps, and 1660 Ω for 100 cps. The filter can be constructed by connecting a capacitor in series with a re-

[5]Sources of such filters include Allison Laboratories, La Habra, California; White Instrument Laboratories, Austin, Texas.

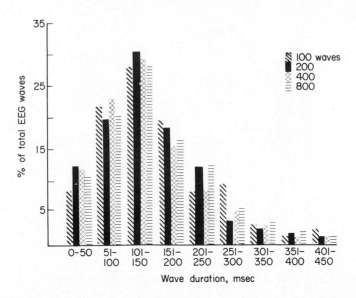

FIG. 5-12.   Interval histogram computed from the same electrode pair on a lightly anesthetized normal dog. All the sample sizes chosen produce about the same interval distributions. (Klemm, 1968a.)

sistor and an alternating current source; output voltage is led off from across the capacitor. The ratio of voltages across the resistor and across the capacitor will determine how much of the applied voltage is available across the capacitor. If the reactance of the capacitor is much lower than the resistance of the resistor, output voltage at the relevant frequencies can be greatly attenuated. If a compounded wave is presented at the input, the output will reveal the same frequencies, but in different voltage ratios. Some frequencies will be barely affected, whereas others will be greatly attenuated, i.e., filtered. In the example cited of leading voltage off the capacitor, high frequencies will be filtered. If the arrangement is reversed with voltages led off the resistor, slow frequencies will be filtered.

The attenuation rate for such RC filters is 6 db (Chapter 4, Section I, C) per octave.[6] This slope is usually not enough. Cascading of identical RC units increases attenuation rate in multiples of 6 db/octave. However, loading interactions occur between successive elements, a problem that can be solved by inserting amplifiers between each RC stage.

[6]This is the interval between 2 frequencies having a ratio of 2:1. For example, one octave from 8 Hz is 16 Hz.

Especially important is a high-impedance input amplifier and a low-impedance output amplifier.

The foregoing discussion is a most elementary form of explanation of electric filtering. Actually, most passive filters also contain inductors, which also impede alternating current. The resistance due to inductance, inductive reactance, behaves in a manner opposite to capacitive reactance, i.e., the higher the frequency, the higher the impedance. In the case of capacitors, the higher the frequency, the lower the impedance.

Selection of the proper inductor and capacitor values, as well as the exact way in which they are connected, is an elaborate and complex art. By appropriate design, a filter can be made to specifically affect any frequency passed through it.

There are certain limitations of passive filters. One problem is that they tend to "ring," that is, produce transient oscillations after receiving an input that rises or falls rapidly. Another problem is the difficulty in designing a good filter for the slow frequencies found in the EEG. The capacitors and inductors required are also inconveniently large. Many problems can be reduced if the EEG is recorded on magnetic tape and the tape played back through filters at a much faster rate. Thus, if one speeds up the time base by a factor of 100, then EEG waves of 1/sec, for example, become 100/sec. This multiplying technique is useful because filters for high frequencies are more reliable and more readily available. It also largely avoids the problem that passive filters produce only graded attenuation of frequencies near the cutoff point, as illustrated in Fig. 5-13.

The design problems, bulkiness, and lack of sharp cutoff with passive filters can be improved by the use of "active" filters,[7] which are specially designed circuits with transistors or tubes. The one problem of such circuits is that they are noisier, by virtue of the active elements; this problem, however, is not serious if the EEG is amplified before filtration. These devices are often used to eliminate one frequency, usually 60 cps, without affecting adjacent frequencies as much as passive filters; for this reason they are often called "notch" filters (Fig. 5-14).

Active filters also provide a more reliable way to filter the slow frequencies present in the EEG. One such filter[8] has been designed to filter out *all* EEG frequencies to permit study of multiple unit (action) potentials from large-diameter, implanted electrodes (Fig. 5-15).

Multiple unit studies have the advantage of statistical averaging—

[7] A. P. Circuit Company, New York, New York; Krohn-Hite Company, Cambridge, Massachusetts; White Instrument Laboratory, Austin, Texas.
[8] David Kopf Instruments, Tujunga, California.

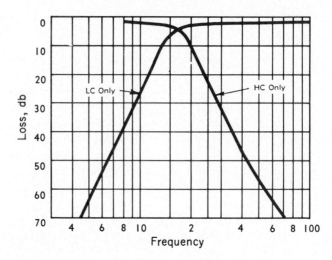

Fɪɢ. 5-13. Sample curves illustrating the extent of attenuation commonly produced by passive filters. LC curve shows attenuation with a filter designed to cut off low frequencies, and HC curve shows the attenuation with a high-frequency cut-off filter.

indicating function of a pool of closely spaced neurons rather than monitoring a single cell, which statistically has very little meaning. There are several ways to quantify multiple unit potentials, one of the more common being integration of the signals (Section III, B, 6). It is also possible to partially separate out action potentials from different units. Separation is made possible by the fact that action potentials from a given cell are usually of the same amplitude at all times at any given distance. The differing amplitudes seen in multiple unit recordings are due to the varying distances of the neurons from the recording electrodes. By using electronic circuits similar to those used in pulse-height analyzers, it is possible to "pick out" only those potentials that have a certain amplitude and thus only those potentials that come from the same cell. Such circuits have preselectable "windows" that disregard all potentials either above or below the threshold values of this window.[9]

Special mention must be made of "frequency analyzers,"[10] which are filters designed to separate the EEG into its various component frequencies (Bickford, 1961; Knott, 1961; Lowenberg and McCullough,

[9]Such an analyzer, specially designed for multiple unit studies, is available from Bio-Medical Electronics, Inc., Rockville, Maryland.

[10]Nihon Kohden Kogyo, Ltd., Tokyo, Japan—U.S. Agent: Lehigh Valley Electronics, Fogelsville, Pennsylvania; San'ei Instrument Company, Tokyo, Japan—U.S. Agent: Medical Systems Corporation, Great Neck, New York.

1963; Shipton, 1961; Walter, 1961). In these devices the EEG is fed simultaneously to a number of different circuits, each adjusted to pick out a different small-frequency band. The output from each filter then can be recorded to reveal the amount of energy present at that frequency in the original EEG. Commonly, such instruments integrate the output in each frequency band and store the output in a storage register, the contents of which drive a special wide-span pen on the original ink record. The integration is carried out over a period of 10 sec and during the next 10 sec the stored data are written out sequentially to form a frequency histogram. This is done by a rotating switch that selects each storage capacitor in turn and allows it to discharge through the ballistic pen. This write-out is usually displayed on the original record of raw data with a 10-sec delay. This display is a series of spikes whose amplitude denoted the "abundance" of a particular frequency band in the period analyzed. Abundance here actually means the integrated voltage of a particular frequency band. During the write-out of an analyzed period, analysis of incoming data continues and the integration during this time is done by using another set of storage capacitors. At the end of 10 sec the role of these capacitors changes from storing a write-out, and the set of capacitors that have been discharged during write-out then become integrators. Another set of capacitors is used to store a fraction of each component and record an average of 4 or 9 analysis periods. A system for producing a digitized average over long periods has been reported (Stern *et al.*, 1963).

The major benefit of such analysis is that it clearly identifies the frequencies present in the compounded EEG. Certain limitations must be recognized, however. For one, the selection of frequency bands is purely arbitrary; also, phase relations are not usually considered.[11] More serious is the emphasis given to amplitude; integration of voltages in each frequency band produces not a simple frequency histogram but a complex misture of frequency and amplitude histogram. This emphasis on amplitude can be inappropriate in certain circumstances. For example, 2 large-amplitude waves in a given band could show more "abundance" upon analysis than 10 low-amplitude waves of the same frequency. Is one justified then in assuming that the 2 waves are more meaningful than the 10 waves? The general comments made previously on the limitations of amplitude analysis also are appropriate here.

Another problem is that the amount of activity in a given band may fluctuate widely with time. Matoušek (1968) proposes a method that

---

[11]Eidelberg and Cheshire (1965) have devised a phase-sensitive analyzer.

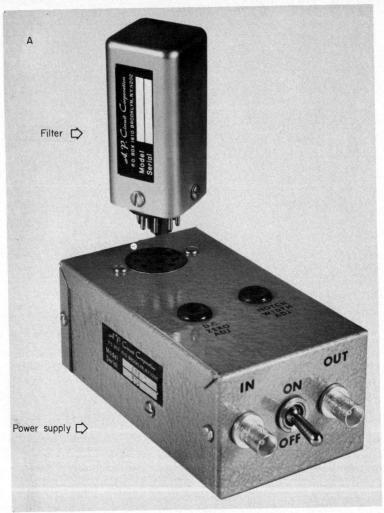

A

Filter ⟹

Power supply ⟹

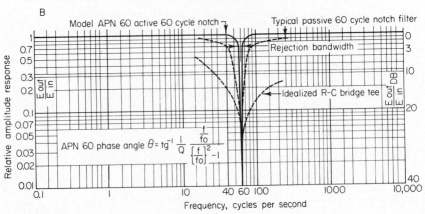

B

Model APN 60 active 60 cycle notch ⟹   Typical passive 60 cycle notch filter

Rejection bandwidth

$\frac{E_{out}}{E_{in}}$

Idealized R-C bridge tee ⟸

APN 60 phase angle $\theta = tg^{-1} \dfrac{1}{Q} \dfrac{\frac{f}{f_0}}{\left[\frac{f}{f_0}\right]^2 - 1}$

Relative amplitude response

$\frac{E_{out}}{E_{in}}$ DB

Frequency, cycles per second

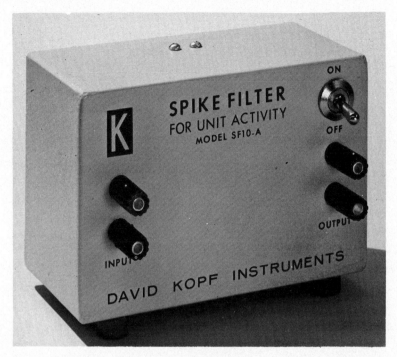

FIG. 5-15. Spike filter that attenuates EEG frequencies and permits recording of multiple unit action potentials from macroelectrodes. (Courtesy of David Kopf Instruments Company.)

compensates for such variability. In principle, the idea is to evaluate the analyzer output in terms of the *ratio* of activity of certain bands of interest; in his study of human theta–alpha ratios, a correction factor was needed.

A final problem is that some very significant waves, like spikes, do not occur often enough and with enough area under their curves to produce much reaction in the analyzer. The analyzer would not be sensitive to their detection and therefore could give misleading information.

4. Auto- and Cross-Correlation

More use of these techniques (Adey, 1961; Barlow, 1961; Kamp *et al.*, 1965; van Leeuwen, 1961) can be expected, because instruments are

---

FIG. 5-14. A: Active "notch" filter for 60 Hz. B: Frequency–response curves showing comparison with passive filter performance. (Courtesy of A. P. Circuit Corporation.)

now commercially available.[12] The techniques permit statistical comparison of spontaneous, as opposed to evoked, EEG signals. Cross correlation compares the frequency content between 2 different EEG signals, whereas autocorrelation compares one signal with a time-displaced version of itself.

Complete understanding of correlation requires mathematical presentations (Lee, 1960) beyond the scope of this book. The basic principles, however, can be stated in words, as has been done in the publication of Anstey (1966).

The aim of EEG correlation is to compare 2 EEG traces. This can be done, as shown in Fig. 5-16, by multiplying discrete samples of voltage values of one trace with corresponding values from the other trace ($p1 \times q1$; $p2 \times q2$; etc.). Then each product is added to arrive at a single number, which is a measure of the similarity between the traces.

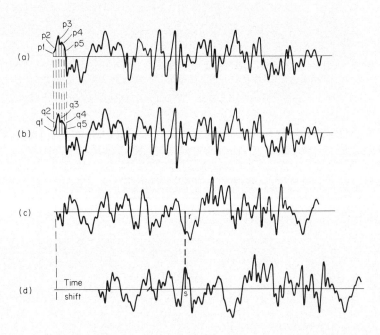

FIG. 5-16.   Hypothetical EEG traces illustrating calculation of correlograms. The top 2 waveforms are identical in shape and phase. The bottom 2 traces are identical in shape, but d is a time-shifted version of c. At a given time, the similarity between voltages in a and b is large while that between b and c or between c and d is small. (Anstey, 1966.)

[12]Princeton Applied Research Corporation, Princeton, New Jersey.

In the example of the figure, the identical nature of traces a and b permits the values, positive or negative, to contribute positive terms to the sum; the sum thus is quite large. However, if such summing were performed on traces made out of phase by time shifting, as between b and c, positive products would tend to be offset by negative products, resulting in a small sum that indicates dissimilarity.

Autocorrelation is illustrated with the traces c and d, which are identical except that d is shifted in time. At that degree of time shift, multiplying ordinate values (such as r and s) produces a small sum because of offsetting positive and negative products. With zero time shift, the sum is large. Time shifting is the key distinction of correlation analysis from frequency analysis. Analysis is said to be in the "time domain" rather than in the "frequency domain."

Actual construction of an autocorrelation curve is illustrated in Fig. 5-17. Here the center section of the diagram illustrates the zero time shift condition where each wave is exactly in phase. At zero time shift, ordinate products are all positive and the sum therefore is large. The left and right sections of the diagram illustrate the situation at a time shift that is equal, but in opposite directions. Some of the ordinate products are positive and others are negative; the sums therefore are small.

In practice, the EEG is correlated during a continuous series of time shifts. If an EEG trace has a high incidence of a repetitive event, autocorrelation will show high values at the time shift (and whole multiples of it) that corresponds to the duration of the repetitive event. This can be made quite obvious by drawing 2 rows of spikes on graph paper, with the same interval between each spike. Then as one row is moved laterally with respect to the other, it is apparent that high correlation values will only occur as the second row is time-shifted to distance equal to the interspike interval. This characteristic of autocorrelation makes it very sensitive for detecting hidden periodicities from a given brain area's activity.

Similar time shifting of 2 different waveforms produces a cross correlation. In Fig. 5-18 we can visualize the lower waveform moving in time past the stationary upper waveform from right to left; then, if correlation is made during the analysis interval ("window of width T"), the sum of multiplied ordinate values will produce values as the function of time shift between them. The practical value of cross correlation lies in its ability to measure similarity between activity from 2 different brain areas, which in turn indicates the degree of functional interdependence between these areas.

A major limitation of all correlation analyses is their dependence upon

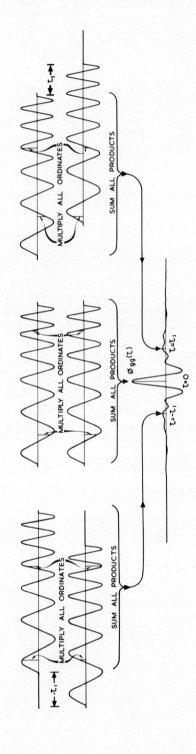

Fig. 5-17.   Sine waves illustrating the process of constructing the autocorrelogram (bottom trace in center). (Anstey, 1966.)

154

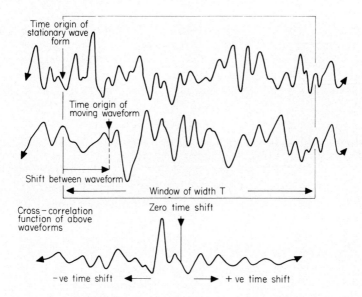

Fɪɢ. 5-18.   Hypothetical EEGs (top 2 traces) illustrating calculation of the cross correlogram. Bottom EEG is time-shifted. The bottom record is the cross correlogram; the maximum in it shows that at that degree of time shift there is a marked similarity between the waveforms, even though this is barely apparent to the eye. (Anstey, 1966.)

amplitude parameters and their inability to distinguish among voltage, frequency, or phase as causes of dissimilarities.

5. *Evoked Response Averaging*

Stimulation of sensory receptors causes evoked responses in the brain (M. H. Goldstein, 1961). Study of these responses, their latency and waveform, yields important information about the input pathways involved in a given sense modality. Such an approach is also useful for mapping neuronal connections within the central nervous system.

The problem of analysis is that the magnitude of the response is often very small, because it originates from a relatively few neurons, and the majority of adjacent neurons generate differing and random potentials which are large, masking the evoked response.

The original technique of analysis consisted of photographing a series of evoked waves displayed on an oscilloscope (Dawson, 1947). The technique requires perfect triggering synchronization and a persistently open shutter. The light beam is made very faint so that random activity is barely perceptible, but repetitive activity that is time-locked to the stimulus (i.e., the evoked response) grows more intense as traces superimpose. The technique has an added advantage in showing variation among responses to the same stimulation.

Special purpose digital computers with built-in programs are available to perform this function[13] (Fig. 5-19). Although these units differ in detail, the basic scheme is about the same. A triggering pulse from the stimulator activates sampling. The analog-to-digital converter in the computer samples the EEG at various times and deposits in the memory electronic pulses that are proportional to the sampled voltage. As each additional stimulus is presented to the animal, results are again recorded at the identical intervals and are added to the results already in the memory. These sums are displayed sequentially on the computer oscilloscope screen. Thus the sum of the responses can be viewed at all times.

As the number of responses increases, all random variations tend to average toward zero, and the time-locked repetitive pattern, the evoked response, will add and become magnified (Fig. 5-20). Random activity cancels because of algebraic addition of voltages of opposite polarity; there is an equal probability for the voltage to be positive or negative at a given instant. Thus, one should expect an increase in the number of responses analyzed to improve the cancellation of background "noise" and to improve the magnification of the evoked response.

Evoked response data can be "read out" of the memory in various ways, either by viewing on the screen, by typed digital data, by plotting on a strip-chart recorder, or by magnetic or paper tape that can be fed into other computers.

6. Integration

Integration is the mathematical determination of the area under a curve. In the case of the EEG, measurements are taken of the entire linear course of each individual wave with concurrent measurement of the area subtended to the zero voltage line or to some arbitrary reference point. Inasmuch as the EEG is a voltage plot as a function of time, such integrated data actually correspond to the electric power content of the EEG.

An ordinary planimeter can achieve the desired integration, but this approach is tedious and time-consuming. Electronic integration is much more effective; the efficiency permits analysis of long segments of EEG

---

[13]Digital Equipment Corporation, Maynard, Massachusetts; Fabri-Tek, Inc., Madison, Wisconsin; Nuclear Chicago, Des Plains, Illinois; Nuclear Data, Inc., Madison, Wisconsin; and Technical Measurements, Inc., North Haven, Connecticut.

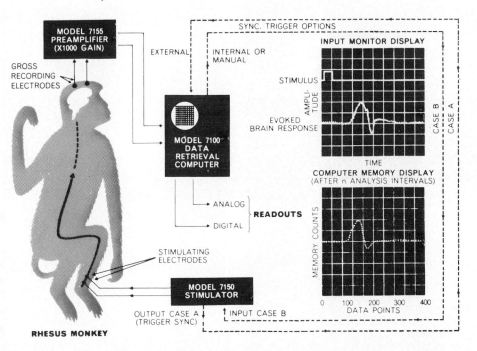

Fig. 5-19. Experimental setup for transient averaging of brain responses evoked by peripheral stimulation. "Data points" refer to a preselected analysis period, divided into 400 time intervals. (Courtesy of Nuclear-Chicago Corporation.)

waves. The classic electronic integrator is simply a capacitor that is charged by incoming signals through a resistor. The surface area of the capacitor determines how much charge can be stored, and the resistance of the resistor determines the rate at which current can flow into and out of the capacitor. Such a resistor–capacitor (RC) integrator produces an output proportional to the average level of the signal at any given time. Adjustable time constant settings can regulate the time required for the integrator to respond to a change of activity, but the "memory time" still is usually less than a few seconds. Another type of integrator cumulatively integrates ("true" integration) the area under the voltage–time curve. Such an integrator has a long memory time yet is still able to respond to instantaneous changes in activity.

Integration of both positive and negative halves of a wave with a zero reference point yields a net value of zero. Thus it is necessary to rectify incoming signals before integration. This requirement simultaneously produces one of the major disadvantages of the integrator methods, namely, that information about polarity is lost. Other serious limitations

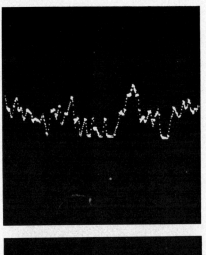

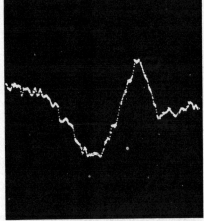

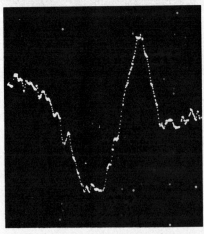

Fig. 5-20. Illustration depicting growth of an evoked response during averaging. Shown are memory contents of computer after successively greater numbers of averages (bottom to top) of cortical responses to sciatic nerve stimulation. (Courtesy of Nuclear-Chicago Corporation.)

are that the technique neglects such parameters as frequencies and phase relations.

The cumulative integrator used by L. Goldstein and Beck (1965) is designed so that each time a capacitor reaches a peak charge, it discharges and simultaneously triggers an output pulse; thus each pulse represents a definite amount of electric energy. Because the data are expressed as pulses, they can be subjected to conventional statistical analyses (Fig. 5-21). In fact, because this is an averaging method, maximum information can be obtained only by statistical analysis of large numbers of successive segments of the EEG.

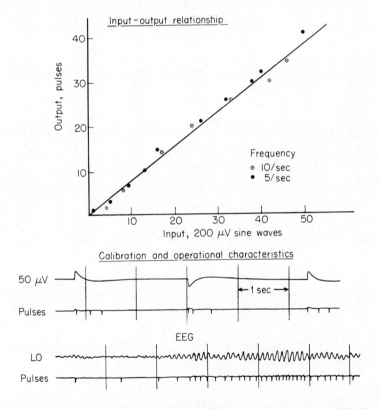

FIG. 5-21. Mode of operation of the Drohocki integrator. Upper graph: Relations between energy input (number of 200 μV sine waves) and integrator output (number of pulses). Despite variation of frequency of the sine waves, the curve is linear. Lower graphs: Calibration and actual integration of a 6-sec strip of left occipital (LO) EEG from a normal human. The standard 50 μV calibration signal corresponds to 3 pulses regardless of polarity (full-wave rectification). (L. Goldstein and Beck, 1965.)

Interpretation of such data in terms of EEG synchrony and desynchrony is relatively straightforward, at least in an oversimplified way. A large number of pulses per second indicates hypersynchrony, because such EEGs usually have high voltage that leads to a more rapid charge buildup on the capacitor, which in turn leads to a more rapid saturation and discharge of pulses. Conversely, a low number of pulses per second indicates desynchrony. Numerous studies have been conducted that demonstrate these correlations, employing a variety of physiologic conditions and drugs that effect the EEG. On the other hand, this association does not exist in some conditions (Chapters 6 and 7).

7. Toposcopy

This technique, in use since 1947, may improve the precision of EEG diagnosis in animals, as it has in man. However, the required equipment is not commercially available. The method permits visual display of the topography (space patterns) of brain electric activity.

The procedure involves the use of numerous electrodes that carry their signals to separate amplifiers (Shipton, 1963). The amplifiers are constructed to amplify only voltage differences, and consequently frequency shifts, within the electrode array. These differences are registered in each channel as light intensity changes in a small cathode ray tube. The electron beam in each cathode-ray tube sweeps radially, as in a radar receiver, with a sweep rate controlled externally or by the brain itself.

Since in-phase activity at the electrodes is suppressed and out-of-phase activity is enhanced, the technique is a useful way to study evoked responses to sensory stimulation. Indeed, one worker froze a small portion of monkey cortex, and with closely spaced electrodes, toposcopy, and a light stimulus localized the epileptic focus and identified its size as 1.5–2 mm.[3]

8. Pattern Recognition

Common patterns observed in EEGs include such things as certain rhythms (theta rhythm), abnormal paroxysms (seizure episodes), or burst activity (spindles). Detection of these and other patterns is most conveniently accomplished by the "eyeball" method. In fact, this is one aspect of human evaluation that is difficult to duplicate by computers.

There are automatic ways to detect certain patterns. For example, the percentage of time an EEG contains a certain rhythm can be calculated with the aid of filters that reject all frequencies besides the ones of interest. Isolated phenomena, such as abnormal paroxysms or spindles, can be automatically quantified by properly programming a computer. For example, the program may direct rejection of all amplitudes below a certain level and all waves of certain frequencies. For burst activity, the program also should reject all wave sequences that do not include the arbitrary number of waves to qualify as a burst. The data thus obtained can be expressed in several ways, such as the number of phenomena per unit time or the percentage of the total time occupied by the phenomena or the interval between phenomena or a distribution of burst lengths.

REFERENCES

Adey, W. R. (1961). Use of correlation analysis in EEG studies of conditioning. *Electroencephalog. Clin. Neurophysiol.* Suppl. 20, 41–48.

Anstey, N. A. (1966). Correlation techniques—a review. *J. Can. Soc. Explor. Geophys.* **2**, 55–82.

Barlow, J. S. (1961). Autocorrelation and crosscorrelation techniques in EEG analysis. *Electroencephalog. Clin. Neurophysiol.* Suppl. 20, 31–36.

Barthel, C. A. (1961). The average reference electrode. *Am. J. EEG Technol.* **1**, 61–74.

Bickford, R. G. (1961). Scope and limitations of frequency analysis. *Electroencephalog. Clin. Neurophysiol.* Suppl. 20, 9–13.

Brazier, M. A. B. (1961). Introductory comments. *Electroencephalog. Clin. Neurophysiol.* Suppl. 20, 2–6.

Bureš, J., Petran, M., and Zachar, J., eds. (1967). "Electrophysiological Methods in Biological Research," 3rd rev. ed. Academic Press, New York.

Dawson, G. D. (1947). Cerebral responses to electrical stimulation of peripheral nerve in man. *J. Neurol., Neurosurg. Psychiat.* [N.S.] **10**, 134–140.

Eidelberg, E., and Cheshire, F. C. (1965). Spectrum analyzer for EEG. *Electroencephalog. Clin. Neurophysiol.* **18**, 85–87.

Ertl, J. P. (1965). Detection of evoked potentials by zero crossing analysis. *Electroencephalog. Clin. Neurophysiol.* **18**, 630–631.

Gibbs, F. A., and Gibbs, E. L. (1964). Exclusive monopolar recordings. *Am. J. EEG Technol.* **4**, 8–9.

Goldstein, M. H. (1961). Averaging techniques applied to evoked responses. *Electroencephalog. Clin. Neurophysiol.* Suppl. 20, 59–63.

Goldstein, L., and Beck, R. A. (1965). Amplitude analysis of the electroencephalogram. *Intern. Rev. Neurobiol.* 8, 265–312.

Jasper, H. H. (1958). The ten twenty electrode system of the international federation. *Electroencephalog. Clin. Neurophysiol.* **10**, 371–375.

Kagawa, N. (1962). Electroencephalography in infants with special reference to the newborn: Technique. *Am. J. EEG Technol.* **2**, 99–105.

Kamp, A., van Leeuwen, W. S., and Tielen, A. M. (1965). A method for auto- and cross-relation analysis of the EEG. *Electroencephalog. Clin. Neurophysiol.* **19**, 91–95.

Klemm, W. R. (1966). Electroencephalographic-behavioral dissociations during animal hypnosis. *Electroencephalog. Clin. Neurophysiol.* **21**, 365–372.

Klemm, W. R. (1968a). Subjective and quantitative analyses of the electroencephalogram of anesthetized normal dogs—control data for clinical diagnosis. *Am. J. Vet. Res.* **29**, 1267–1277.

Klemm, W. R. (1968b). Attempts to standardize veterinary electroencephalographic techniques. *Am. J. Vet. Res.* **29**, 1895–1900.

Knott, J. R. (1961). Some comments on automatic low frequency analysis. *Electroencephalog. Clin. Neurophysiol.* Suppl. 20, 22–24.

Lee, Y. W. (1960). "Statistical Theory of Communication." Wiley, New York.

Lowenberg, E. C., and McCullough, C. E. (1963). An improved HI-Q band-pass filter for electroencephalography. *Electroencephalog. Clin. Neurophysiol.* **15**, 706–708.

Maloney, J. V., and Bradham, G. B. (1965). Computers in medicine. *Ann. Rev. Med.* **16**, 239–252.

Marshall, C. (1955). An EEG Ruler. *Electroencephalog. Clin. Neurophysiol.* **7**, 310.

Matousek, M. (1968). Frequency analysis in routine electroencephalography. *Electroencephalog. Clin. Neurophysiol.* **24**, 365–373.

Mavor, H., and Hellen, M. K. (1964). Nasopharyngeal electrode recording. *Am. J. EEG Technol.* **4**, 43–50.

Mowery, G. L., and Bennett, A. E. (1961). Some technical notes on monopolar and bipolar recording. *Am. J. EEG Technol.* **1**, 31–41.

Pampiglione, G. (1956). Some anatomical considerations upon electrode placement in routine E. E. G. *Proc. Electro-Physiol. Tech. Assoc.* **7**, 1–11.

Rosenblith, W. A. (1962). "Processing Neuroelectric Data." M.I.T. Press, Cambridge, Massachusetts.

Sheatz, G. C. (1964). An inclined plane magnifying ruler for EEG Y axis measurement. *Electroencephalog. Clin. Neurophysiol.* **16**, 524–525.

Shipton, H. W. (1961). Engineering considerations in the design of wave-form analyzers of the Walter-type. *Electroencephalog. Clin. Neurophysiol.* Suppl. 20, 25–30.

Shipton, H. W. (1963). A new frequency-selective toposcope for electroencephalography. *Med. Electron. Biol. Eng.* **1**, 483–495.

Stern, J. A., Durham, J., and Loeffel, R. (1963). Trials and tribulations in automating the output of a frequency analyzer. *Am. J. EEG Technol.* **3**, 83–89.

Suckling, E. E. (1961). "Bioelectricity." McGraw-Hill, New York.

Turner, W. J. (1955). An electroencephalographic ruler. *Electroencephalog. Clin. Neurophysiol.* **7**, 309.

Ulam, S. M. (1964). Computers. *Sci. Am.* **211**, 203–216.

van Leeuwen, W. S. (1961). Comparison of EEG data obtained with frequency analysis and with correlation methods. *Electroencephalog. Clin. Neurophysiol.* Suppl. 20, 37–40.

Walter, W. G. (1961). Frequency analysis. *Electroencephalog. Clin. Neurophysiol.* Suppl. 20, 9–13.

Walter, W. G. (1963). Technique-interpretation. *In* "Electroencephalography" (J. D. N. Hill and G. Parr, eds.), pp. 65–98. Macmillan, New York.

6

EEG Correlates of Physiologic Changes

I. Maturation of the EEG

The brain of newborn animals is neither structurally nor functionally fully developed; in particular, many studies have demonstrated post-natal maturation processes in cerebral cortex. The neural immaturity of the newborn is reflected in the EEG. During the first few hours of life in kittens, for example, the EEG is mainly isoelectric. The EEG develops quickly after birth; during sleep of 1-week-old kittens, the EEG reveals low voltage, fast activity (LVFA) about 90% of the time (refer to para-doxical sleep, Section II, C, 1). During the second week, more varia-bility appears in the EEG, showing some LVFA during wakefulness and some high voltage, slow activity (HVSA) and "spindles" (Section II, C, 1) during sleep. At 3 weeks, the EEG resembles that of the adult, with a greater incidence of distinct slow waves during sleep (Valtax *et al.*, 1964; Fig. 6-1). Studies conducted during barbiturate anesthesia (Grossman, 1955) revealed qualitatively similar EEGs, except that adult-type spon-taneous activity was not obtained until about the tenth week. Anesthetic studies in dogs by Fox (1964) revealed similar results and emphasized that cortical EEGs were flat during the first 3 weeks. The study of un-anesthetized dogs by Pampiglione (1963) revealed frequent isoelectric periods during the first week of life, followed by a progressive develop-ment of activity with age. A mature EEG developed at about 5 months, consisting of posterior 6–8/sec waves, interrupted by 12–14/sec rhythms and faster irregular activity. EEG responses to stimuli developed after the first 3–3½ weeks of age. Sleep spindles began to appear at about 2 months of age.

Similar findings have been reported in other species; however, the time course varies, commonly depending upon the expected life span

163

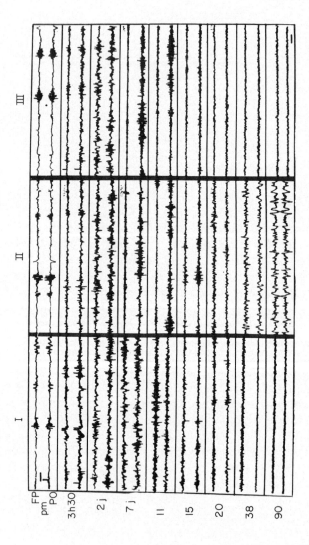

FIG. 6-1. Maturation of the cat's EEG from birth to 90 days in various behavioral states. I: Awake; II: light sleep; and III: paradoxical sleep (PS). At each age the upper trace is derived from the region of the coronal suture; the second, from the occipital region. pm: premature kitten (weight = 50 gm). In the first days [3½ hours, 2 days (2j)], the EEG did not differ much during the 3 behavioral states. Beginning about the seventh day (7j). LVFA appeared during PS. At about the fifteenth day, EEG arousal patterns of LVFA occurred during wakefulness. At about the twentieth day, HVSA appeared during light sleep, and it developed progressively with increasing age. (Valtax *et al.*, 1964.)

of individuals in a given species. Guinea pigs, for example, exhibit distinct EEG activity *in utero* during the forty-sixth to sixtieth day of gestation (Flexner *et al.*, 1950; Jasper *et al.*, 1937). Newborn rabbits, cats, and dogs reveal a predominant low voltage EEG, which within 2–8 days becomes HVSA during sleep (Petersen *et al.*, 1964). Sleep spindles develop about 1–3 weeks later in rabbits and cats and about 6–8 weeks later in dogs. Paradoxical sleep and its concomitant EEG of LVFA develop at about 1 week in rabbits and at about 2 weeks in cats and dogs. Monkeys at 4 days of age exhibit a flattened EEG, with normal adult-type patterns appearing at about 2 years (Kennard and Nims, 1942). Humans do not develop adult EEGs until 10–12 years.

Responsiveness of the cortex to intense stimulation also changes with age. Newborn rats, for example, are not able to develop convulsions in response to intense electric shock (Heim, 1967). In newborn rabbits, cortical excitation with direct current or KCl has little effect, whereas such stimulation in rabbits over 1 month of age causes EEG isoelectric activity (Schadé and Pascoe, 1964; Fig. 6-2); this response is called "spreading depression" because it spreads from a focus to involve more and more cortex (Bureš *et al.*, 1967).

Other indicators of responsivity are evoked cortical responses to sensory stimulation. Latency of evoked potentials of dogs attain mature characteristics between 5–6 weeks of age (Fox, 1967). In anesthetized cats, evoked potentials become of the mature type at around 10 weeks (Grossman, 1955).

II. Behavioral Correlates

Unless otherwise stated, the following commentary applies specifically to adult mammals.

A. Alert Wakefulness

The EEG of normal, unanesthetized cats has been well described by Bradley and Elkes (1957). In the fully alert state the EEG amplitude is at a minimum. No dominant rhythms are present; rather, a wide spectrum of frequencies exists, usually in the range of about 15–30/sec. In the resting or relaxed state, HVSA becomes apparent, along with spindles that take the form of bursts of 5–8/sec activity with amplitudes of up to 200 μV. The HVSA becomes more prominent during drowsiness, with slow waves of 1–3/sec and amplitudes of up to 500 μV. Spindles of 12–15/sec activity are also more prominent as drowsiness progresses.

The basic scheme just outlined applies in general to all higher animals.

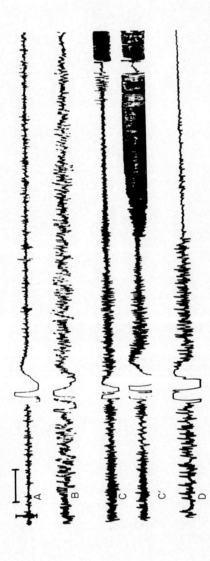

FIG. 6-2.   Spreading depression and spreading convulsion during maturation of rabbits. A: Cortical stimulation (10 V, DC) for 3 sec in 8-day-old rabbit; B: cortical stimulation (12 V, DC) for 3 sec in 15-day-old rabbit; C and C′: cortical stimulation (10 V, DC) for 3 sec in 24-day-old rabbit, C′ recording from electrodes closest to stimulus and C recording from more caudal electrodes; and D: cortical stimulation (6 V, DC) for 3 sec in adult rabbit, D recording from electrodes closest to stimulus. All preparations were lightly anesthetized with urethan. Stimuli are recognizable by stimulus artifacts. Calibrations: 1 mV; 10 sec. (Schade and Pascoe, 1964.)

There are species differences, but these have not been well studied nor quantified. There are also differences in the EEG among animals within a given species; these differences are minor and do not lend themselves well to description. In any event, we can generally characterize the EEG of all higher animals as LVFA (during alertness) and as HVSA (during drowsiness). Within a given animal, EEG voltages and frequencies are very consistent under consistent environmental conditions. For example, I have recorded from unanesthetized rabbits under constant conditions over a 14-day period and found that, although there were minor differences among different animals, the EEG was remarkably constant within a given animal, both cortically and subcortically (Klemm, 1963).

When an animal is relaxed and is presented with a novel or biologically significant stimulus, the cortical EEG changes from HVSA to LVFA; such a response is often called an "arousal response" (Fig. 6-3). This LVFA is sometimes referred to as desynchrony. The term is derived from the hypothesis that a synchronous waveform, such as HVSA, results from summation of membrane potential (MP) oscillations in parallel reverberating circuits that are firing synchronously. Such synchronous reverberation would be expected to produce a high voltage because of summation of in-phase potentials. The slower frequencies observed during HVSA arise in part from voltage summation and may also be related to more temporal and spatial summation in the synchronized generation of MP fluctuations (Chapter 1).

EEG desynchrony during behavioral arousal is supposedly produced by intense afferent input that disrupts smooth reverberating firing and produces rapid MP changes. The physiologic mechanisms by which desynchrony is produced include the neural activating functions of the ascending reticular arousal system (ARAS) in the brain stem (Fig. 6-4). This system receives collateral sensory input from all major sensory channels and projects an excitatory drive diffusely upon the cortex (reviewed by Rossi and Zanchetti, 1957; Klemm, 1969). The EEG arousal response parallels a simultaneous behavioral arousal and is a reflection of the processes by which an animal becomes attentive to stimuli and responds appropriately.

There are certain conditions in normal animals in which arousing stimuli fail to produce cortical desynchrony. These usually are pre-existing desynchrony states or conditions of accommodation, wherein repeated delivery of the stimulus eventually loses its biologic significance and the animal no longer responds to it, behaviorally or physiologically.

Several interesting and uncommon phenomena occur in the EEG of alert frogs (Hobson, 1957a,b). EEGs, especially in frontal regions, consistently show a HVSA during alertness that is due to olfactory evoked potentials (Figs. 6-5 and 6-6). Both the synchrony and respiratory rate directly relate to the amount of general behavioral activity. Synchrony stops when frogs stop breathing. During rapid breathing, synchrony is continuous. As final proof that the synchrony is not artifact, cutting the olfactory bulbs prevents respiration-induced synchrony without affecting respiration.

These frog studies also indicated that frogs were in a continual state of wakefulness. Even during immobility, the EEG was desynchronized; Hobson concludes that frogs do not sleep. Although the dream stage of sleep in higher animals coexists with a desynchronized EEG, frogs did

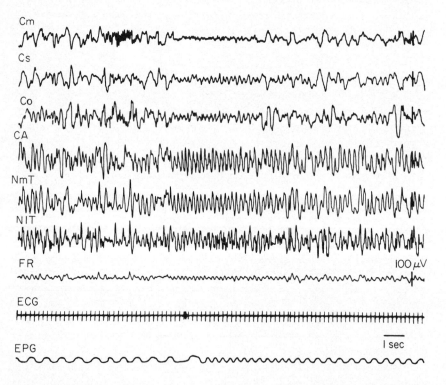

FIG. 6-3. Spontaneous brain electric activity of the unanesthetized rabbit when relaxed (beginning and end of record) and when excited (middle of record). Simultaneous recording of pulse rate (ECG) and respiration (EPG). The arousal reaction consists of LVFA in the motor cortex, some tendency toward a theta rhythm in other cortical regions, and definite theta rhythms in the subcortical regions. Acceleration of respiration also accompanies arousal. Cm: Motor cortex; Cs: sensory cortex; Co: occipital cortex; CA: cornu ammonis (hippocampus); NmT: nucleus medial thalamus; NlT: nucleus lateral thalamus; and FR: reticular formation. (Monnier and Gangloff, 1961.)

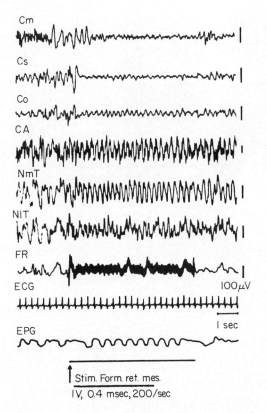

Cm

Cs

Co

C A

NmT

NlT

FR

ECG   100 μV

                                          I sec

EPG

Stim. Form. ret. mes.
I V, 0.4 msec, 200/sec

FIG. 6-4. Production of the cortical and subcortical arousal reactions by high-frequency stimulation in an unanesthetized rabbit of the midbrain reticular formation beginning at arrow (Stim. Form. ret. mes.). Symbols identifying brain areas are the same as in Fig. 6-3. (Monnier and Gangloff, 1961.)

not display any other signs of dream sleep, such as twitching or rapid eye movements.

What changes occur in brain areas other than the cortex during arousal? This question is not easy to answer, because activity can differ widely among the various subcortical regions. Activity in many regions does parallel cortical activity. Activity in the amygdala is said to change to an increased amount of high voltage, *fast* activity during behavioral arousal (Pagano and Gault, 1964; Fig. 6-7). The most dependable and conspicuous electrographic response, at least in nonprimates, is the onset of a synchronous 4–7/sec "theta" rhythm during cortical desynchrony (Figs. 6-3 and 6-4). This theta rhythm is found in most parts of the limbic system, especially the hippocampus (Green and Arduini, 1954). Rabbits, which have a large amount of limbic cortex, present a

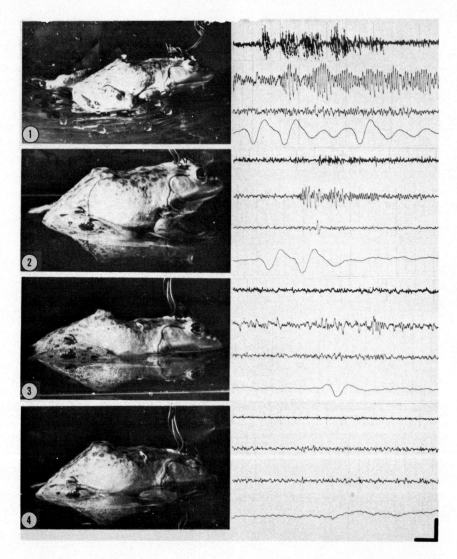

FIG. 6-5.   Photographs of a frog in each of 4 behavioral states. 1: Activity (walking); 2: sitting; 3: reclining; and 4: withdrawal. To the right of each photograph are examples of corresponding electrographic data: upper channel, EMG (electromyogram); second channel, frontal EEG; third channel, occipital EEG; and fourth channel, respiration. Throat movement alone is indicated in the top respiratory record by 4 smaller amplitude sinusoidal deflections and compound throat and flank movements by the 3 larger amplitude notched deflections. This segment of record would give a respiratory ratio of 3/7. In the other tracings shown, only combined movements are recorded. Note the tendency of the rate of flank movement and EEG amplitude and rhythmicity to increase together with physical activity. Calibrations: 20 μV (for EEG and EMG); 1 sec. (Hobson, 1967a.)

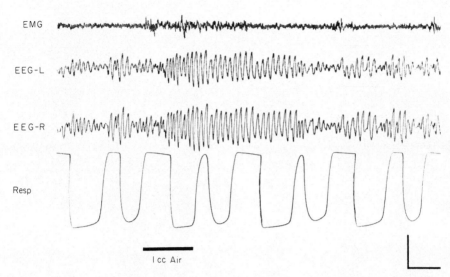

EMG

EEG-L

EEG-R

Resp

I cc Air

FIG. 6-6. Train of synchronous waves (from left and right hemispheres, EEG-L, EEG-R) induced by injection of air into the nasal cavity of frogs. The time of the air stimulus is approximately indicated by the solid black line under the tracings. Note that the background activity is synchronous in relation to a one-to-one throat-to-flank pattern of respiration and can be seen to interact with the evoked response. Calibrations: 25 μV; 1 sec. (Hobson, 1967b.)

special case in that sometimes arousing stimuli produce a theta rhythm in the cortex as well as in the hippocampus (Fig. 6-8). Another interesting aspect of theta rhythm is that, at least in the hippocampus, the large waves mask a smaller voltage, fast-frequency component of 40–60/sec (Stumpf, 1965).

One of the theories for the cause of synchronous theta activity is that inhibitory neurons may act as pacemakers by periodically inhibiting activity in ascending afferent pathways (Eccles, 1964). Considerable evidence exists that these pacemaker cells are located in the septum (reviewed by Stumpf, 1965).

Recent discoveries that cortical LVFA is not always accompanied by limbic theta rhythms have opened important new areas of physiologic investigations (Lena and Parmeggiani, 1964). Under conditions of *intense* stimulation of the ARAS of cats, hippocampal theta rhythm converts to LVFA without any apparent change in the existing cortical LVFA (Stumpf, 1965). Lesions in the limbic system cause animals to become excessively alert, accompanied by hippocampal LVFA (Lena and Parmeggiani, 1964). Such evidence has led to a hypothesis of 2 systems associated with behavioral and EEG arousal, the ARAS and the limbic system.

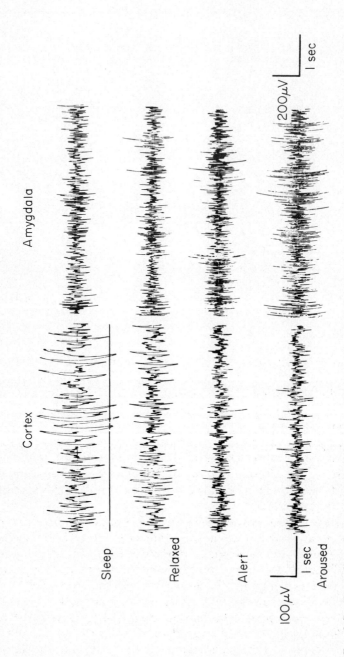

Fig. 6-7. Recordings from a cat illustrating amygdaloid and cortical activity for each behavioral category. Cortical recordings are bipolar; amygdaloid traces are recorded with a reference electrode. There is an increase in amygdala large-amplitude fast activity and a corresponding decrease in cortical slow activity as the subject's activation level changes from sleep to arousal. (Pagona and Gault, 1964.)

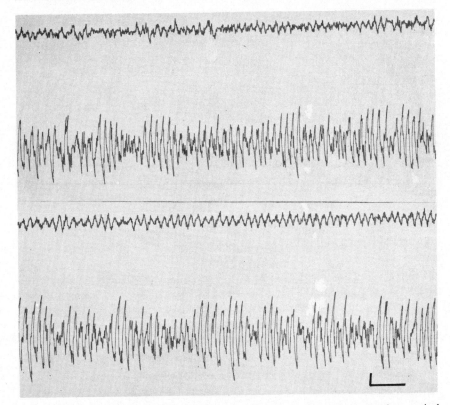

FIG. 6-8. Two types of arousal patterns that occur in alert rabbits, showing cortical (upper trace of each pair) desynchrony (upper half of figure) or theta rhythm (lower half of figure) during apparently identical behavior states. Theta rhythm in dorsal hippocampus (lower trace of each pair) remains essentially unchanged. Calibrations: 50 μV; 1 sec.

Understanding the interactions between these 2 systems and the cerebral cortex eventually may explain previously demonstrated exceptions to the concept that behavioral arousal is associated with cortical LVFA. Several such dissociations between behavior and the EEG have been reported over the years, none of which have been explained. As mentioned, the EEG and behavior are usually associated, in the desynchronized (activated) EEGs occur during behavioral alertness and synchronized (deactivated) EEGs occur during behavioral sedation. Such associations raise important questions about the relative roles of facilitating and inhibiting neural systems.

The fact that dissociation states occur requires us to reexamine more closely the concept of association. Actually, the idea of association is superficial, and a more critical evaluation is needed. For example, there is the question of the role of neural inhibition in the genesis of the EEG. Does an activated EEG, for example, result from facilitatory influences or from disinhibition, or both? Certainly, facilitatory drive from the ARAS promotes cortical desynchrony; the role of active inhibition is much less clear. One visual-response study showed that changes in active inhibition had no gross effect on the occipital EEG (Demetrescu *et al.*, 1966). On the other hand, disinhibition (decreased IPSP activity) seems critical for development of EEG epileptiform activity (Ajmone Marsan, 1965; Chapter 7).

A more obvious problem is the common inexact use of the terms alertness and sedation. Sedation, for example, can refer to decreased sensory input, sensory processing, motor output, or any combination thereof. These considerations have not been critically examined in studies from which conclusions were drawn about EEG-observations of gross motor activity: decreased in sedation; increased in alertness. Such changes may or may not have been paralleled by similar changes in specific sensory or integrative functions. To extend conclusions to sensory functions when they were not specifically studied is unwarranted. Complete understanding requires exploration of these "new" dimensions of the dissociation concept with each known condition of dissociation. With the dissociations we will subsequently consider, relevance to concepts of brain inhibitory functions is reliable only concerning inhibition of integrated motor activity.

The known examples of dissociation can be classified into two major categories. The first of these involves *behavioral alertness with EEG deactivation*. The classic example of such a dissociation is that produced by injection of atropine. Atropine deactivates EEGs coincident with apparent behavioral alertness (Fig. 6-9). This dissociation has since been proved to be only partial; several studies demonstrated that atropine impairs sensory processes. The atropine antagonist, eserine, restores both an activated EEG and sensory function, suggesting parallelism — not dissociation — between EEG and behavior (Longo, 1966).

Another example is the cortical deactivation that can be present in humans shortly after arousal from sleep (reviewed by Prince and Shanzer, 1966). Also, anesthetized normal cats reportedly can respond to intense ARAS stimulation with body movements and apparently lighter stages of anesthesia, accompanied by enhanced cortical deactivation (Prince and Shanzer, 1966).

The second dissociation category is *behavioral sedation with EEG activation*. These states involve motor inhibition, and some evidence suggests

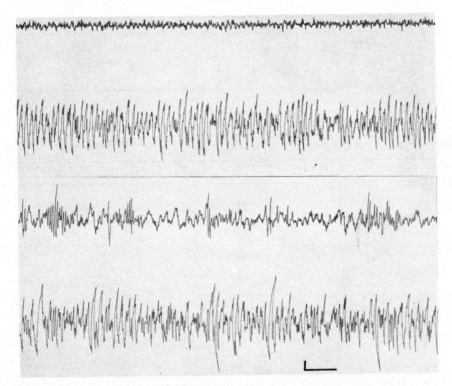

Fig. 6-9. EEG-behavioral dissociation produced by intravenous injection of atropine (2 mg/kg) in a rabbit. Gross behavior before drug (upper pair of traces) was not changed by the drug, although the drug induced cortical synchrony (lower pair of traces). Upper trace in each pair taken from motor cortex; lower trace taken from dorsal hippocampus. Calibrations: 50 μV; 1 sec.

that the motor inhibition is not necessarily paralleled by an equivalent depression of sensory function; unfortunately, little direct evidence is available. Most workers, however, accept the concept that EEG activation represents activation of sensory processes (Moruzzi and Magoun, 1949; Lindsley, 1952; Rossi and Zanchetti, 1957).

Drug-induced dissociations in this category include those caused by reserpine (Pscheidt *et al.*, 1963; Fig. 6-10) and by the administration of eserine to chlorpromazine-treated animals (Bradley and Hance, 1957).

Such dissociations also occur in certain disease states. Some comatose humans with certain brain-stem lesions exhibit an activated EEG (reviewed by Otomo, 1966). I have seen activated EEGs (with desynchrony,

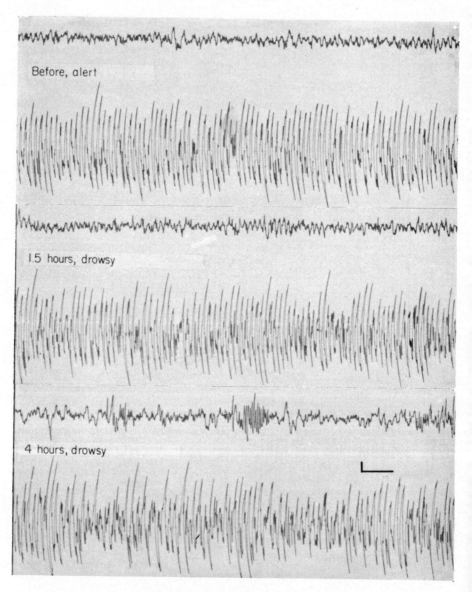

FIG. 6-10.   EEG-behavioral dissociation produced by intramuscular injection of reserpine (1.5 mg/kg) in a rabbit. At the 2 times after injection, the gross behavior was identically that of drowsiness, yet at 1.5 hr the cortical EEG was desynchronized. Upper trace of each pair taken from motor cortex; lower trace taken from the dorsal hippocampus. Calibrations: 50 μV; 1 sec.

spikes, and even electrographic seizures) in many surgically anesthetized dogs with a variety of neurologic disorders (Chapter 7).

Similar dissociations occur in human hypnosis. Hypnotized humans can exhibit activated EEG patterns without parallel changes in motor behavior (Chertok and Kramarz, 1959; Loomis *et al.*, 1936). Similar findings occur in so-called animal hypnosis (Fig. 6-11A). In fact, the dissociation is more drastic than the mere presence of EEG arousal patterns. Electrographic seizures occur spontaneously on rare occasions during hypnosis; moreover, seizures can be induced by drugs, before or during hypnosis, without disrupting the immobility (Klemm, 1966a; Fig. 6-11B).

Another example of dissociation is paradoxical sleep (PS). Motor functions, however, are only partially inhibited because there is phasic activity. Much evidence supports the conclusion that PS involves an active inhibitory process on motor neurons (Pompeiano, 1967). There is little ground to suspect that sensory functions are likewise inhibited. Not only is the EEG activated, but visually evoked responses are more enhanced in PS than during slow-wave sleep (Demetrescu *et al.*, 1966). However, these studies indicated visual facilitatory influences during wakefulness and PS but active inhibitory processes only during alert wakefulness. Thus, EEGs that appear to indicate a similar degree of cortical activation do not necessarily reflect the same degree of cortical excitability. On the other hand, statistical relations involved in the genesis of the EEG suggest that a few sensory circuits could operate independently of the majority without much net effect on the EEG.

In the last year or two, investigators have begun to correlate behavior changes with multiple-unit activity (action potentials derived simultaneously from many neurons). For example, thalamic and ARAS units displayed increased activity during behavioral arousal and PS, whereas that activity decreased during sedation (Podvoll and Goodman, 1967). Similarly, unit activity in the hypothalamus increased during EEG desynchrony and decreased during EEG synchrony; during cortical spindling, the unit activity decreased with occasional surges of increase (Beyer *et al.*, 1967). Such associations are not inevitable, however, because Buchwald *et al.* (1966) found no consistent relation between evoked EEG potentials and unit activity. Acoustical EEG evoked responses in the reticular formation and acoustic nuclei were associated with increased unit activity in those regions but not in other areas, even though EEG changes were evident. A major reason for these discrepancies is that the unit activity recorded comes from both excitatory and inhibitory neurons.

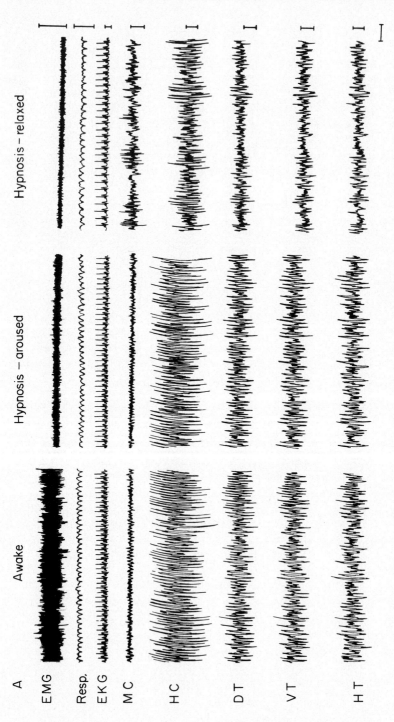

Fig. 6-11. A: Records illustrating physiologic conditions during alert wakefulness and during alert (hypnosis-aroused) and relaxed (hypnosis-relaxed) stages of animal hypnosis. EMG: Electromyogram; RESP.: respiration; EKG: electrocardiogram; MC: motor cortex; HC: hippocampus; DT: dorsal thalamus; VT: ventral thalamus; and HT: hypothalamus. Calibrations: 100 μV; 1 sec. (Klemm, 1966a.)

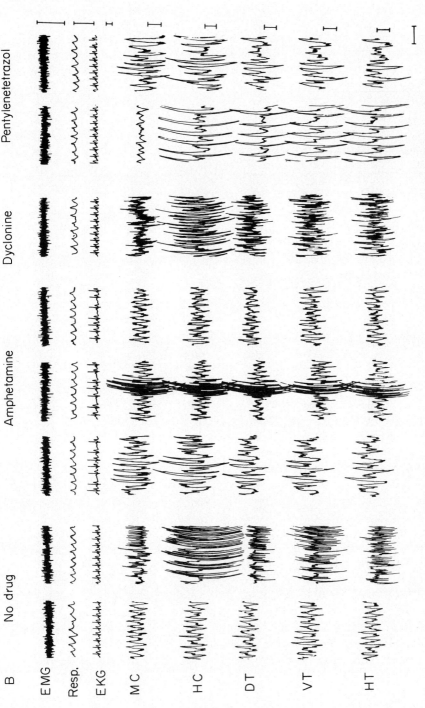

FIG. 6-11.   B: Records illustrating various types of seizure activity in rabbits during hypnosis, with and without drug treatment. Abbreviations are the same as in Part A. Calibrations: 100 μV; 1 sec. (Klemm, 1966a.)

Special attention must be given to the interpretation of unit activity changes. For example, increased unit activity in a pool of neurons may indicate that they were directly activated by afferent input or that they were indirectly activated by removal of inhibitory input (disinhibition). Decreased unit activity may indicate that the neurons were directly inhibited by afferent input or that they were indirectly inhibited by removal of facilitating input (disfacilitation).

Shifts in ultraslow potentials also have been correlated with alertness. During behavioral arousal there is a negative cortical shift relative to an indifferent electrode in bone (Caspers, 1961). A similar shift, but with positive polarity, was reported by Wurtz (1965), who used subcortical white matter as the reference region.

The correlation of such shifts with arousal seems valid, inasmuch as they can be duplicated by direct stimulation of brain reticular formation (Hayward *et al.*, 1966). Superimposed on the shifts in cats are spontaneous slow oscillations, ranging from 0.5 to 12/min, which do not seem to vary consistently with various degrees of alertness (Norton and Jewett, 1965a,b; Fig. 6-12).

B. Conditioned Learning

1. Conditioned Arousal

EEG arousal patterns have been reported in many species during the development of conditioned responses, CR (Wells, 1963). Arousal patterns should be expected because recognition of conditioning stimuli (CS) and performance of CRs requires alert behavior. Many studies have demonstrated that the area of cortex that is desynchronized becomes progressively smaller as training proceeds.

Grastyán *et al.* (1959) found that the first presentation of a CS to cats produced a "startle" response, associated with LVFA in both cortical and hippocampal areas. After several stimulus presentations, a so-called "orienting" response developed, associated with cortical LVFA and and hippocampal theta rhythms. When a stable reflex was established, the EEG arousals disappeared. The initial response of LVFA in the hippocampus was not confirmed, however, in the conditioning studies of Adey *et al.* (1960). The apparent discrepancy might be explained by differences in stimulus intensity. As mentioned before, strong arousal of cats produces hippocampal LVFA, whereas less intense stimuli only produce theta rhythms in the hippocampus.

Conditioning studies often have emphasized the activity of the hippo-

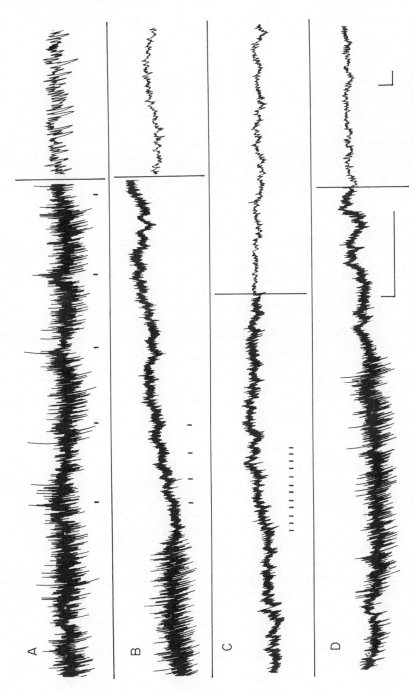

Fig. 6-12.   Spontaneous cortical slow potentials in the cat. A: 1/min waves during light sleep (as indicated by the dots); B: transition from light sleep to PS with negative shift in base line during PS. — slow wave (0.7/min) with 3/min waves superimposed; C: alert cat with 11/min waves; and D: light sleep and PS, both with 1/min waves. Calibrations: on left of vertical line of each record, 200 μV and 1 min; on the right, 200 μV and 1 sec. Negativity up. (Norton and Jewett, 1965a.)

campus, because many lines of evidence point to this structure as important in learning and memory (John, 1967).

EEG arousal responses during conditioning cannot be studied conveniently unless the experimental paradigm permits the animal to have a relaxed EEG pattern. Sometimes this is not possible, and animals are pretreated with bulbocapnine, a drug that produces relaxed EEG patterns without any *known* effects on conditioning behavior. Drug-induced EEG patterns are still capable of changing to alert patterns during conditioning (Beck *et al.*, 1958).

If EEG patterns are alert before conditioning trials, it is sometimes possible to detect changes during training. In the operant conditioning test of rabbits by Sadowski and Longo (1962), rabbits were conditioned to pull a ring with the mouth during the sound of a buzzer in order to obtain food. The EEG prior to sound of the buzzer was of the arousal type. During CS presentation, the hippocampal rhythm increased to frequencies of 8–9/sec with higher amplitude. No cortical changes were evident, except in the few animals whose initial anterior cortex indicated high voltage, fast activity of about 60/sec; this activity abruptly changed to low voltage, 25–30/sec waves during CS presentation (Fig. 6-13).

This study also raised interesting questions about so-called "masticatory" waves of rabbits. Though artifact might be suspected, these waves can disappear during EEG synchrony or desynchrony, even though eating persists. The mechanisms are not understood. Similar masticatory waves occur in goats (Fig. 6-14).

Lip smacking in the rabbit can produce unusual high voltage bursts in the cerebellum and perhaps elsewhere (Fig. 6-15). It is difficult to say whether this represents artifact or is neural potential being generated in the circuits that control the motor act.

Studies also have been devoted to the process termed by Pavlov as "internal inhibition,"[1] a condition usually associated with synchronized EEGs (reviewed by Weinberger *et al.*, 1968). Rowland and Gluck (1960) used a 2/sec click as a CS and an electric skin shock as the unconditioned stimulus (US). Increasing the CS–US interval during training revealed that short delays desynchronized the EEG, but long delays (over 60 sec) did not. The CS produced an initial desynchrony, which quickly

---

[1]"Inhibition" is used in many contexts with different meanings, and the meaning here is perhaps less clear than elsewhere. Internal inhibition refers generally to inhibitory responses that develop with conditioning. We have discussed elsewhere inhibition of individual neurons (postsynaptic and presynaptic), inhibition of pools of neurons, and inhibited behavior.

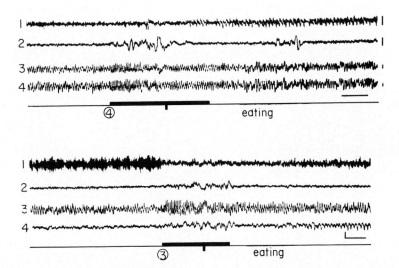

FIG. 6-13. The figure illustrates 2 different EEG patterns observed during an alimentary conditioned reflex. In the upper tracing there is an increase in voltage and in the frequency of the hippocampal waves when the conditioned stimulus was presented with no changes in cortical leads. During the eating period, "masticatory" waves appear in the anterior sensorimotor cortex. The lower tracing shows 60 cps high voltage waves in the anterior sensorimotor cortex (frequency measured in curves recorded at high speed), which disappear when the conditioned stimulus is presented. The modifications of hippocampal activity are similar to those shown in the tracing reproduced above. The horizontal black line indicates the duration of buzzer sounding. The number of the trial is indicated below the line. The vertical mark indicates the rabbit response of pulling the ring. Lead identification: 1, anterior sensorimotor cortex; 2, associative cortex; 3, left dorsal hippocampus; and 4, right dorsal hippocampus (upper tracings) and right ventromedial nucleus of the thalamus (lower tracings). Calibrations: 100 μV (upper tracings) and 200 μV (lower tracings); 2 sec. (Sadowski and Longo, 1962.)

changed to synchrony that persisted for 40–60 sec. Then followed a period of desynchrony that differed from the original desynchrony in that it was less diffuse and some brain areas desynchronized as much as 10 sec before the association cortex did. Subsequent studies have confirmed the internal inhibiting effect during delayed conditioning (Wells, 1963).

One could question whether such synchrony reflects active inhibitory processes or is a simple consequence of decreased attentiveness. One study (Weinberger *et al.*, 1968) supports the decreased attentiveness hypothesis. Vigilant cats, trained to inhibit licking of a food cup, revealed desynchronized EEGs during the inhibition of licking, whereas EEGs were synchronized during general activity inhibition. As the au-

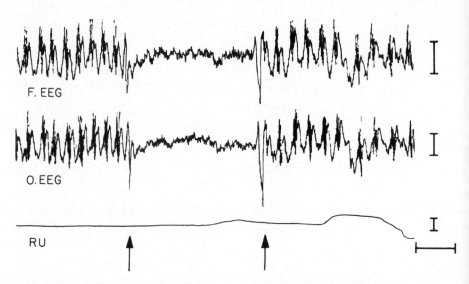

FIG. 6-14. Records illustrating presence of alert EEG patterns when goats are lying quiet and ruminating. The alert EEG patterns that are obscured by chewing potentials become quite distinct during a lapse in rumination. Arrow at left indicates swallowing of bolus; arrow on right indicates regurgitation. F. EEG: Frontal; O. EEG: occipital; and RU: impedance changes of rumen contractions. Calibrations: horizontal line, 2 sec; vertical lines 100 μV (EEG) and 5 Ω (impedance of rumen). (Klemm, 1966b.)

thors point out, the cortical EEG may not be the most sensitive indicator of active inhibition. Especially in aroused animals, other indices of brain activity (ultraslow shifts, amygdala-hippocampal activity, and recruiting responses) may be more sensitive indicators.

Another useful indication of active inhibitory brain functions is obtainable from studies of evoked responses to paired stimuli (Demetrescu et al., 1966), although this technique has not been used in tests of internal inhibition. The basic scheme is to stimulate a sensory path with a pair of pulses (about 7–15 msec apart), followed 50–70 msec later by another pulse pair. Recording the evoked responses in awake cats revealed that the shortly delayed stimuli (second and fourth) yielded suppressed evoked responses that were interpreted as indicating active inhibition. Increases in first and third evoked responses, which occurred in alertness, were interpreted to indicate enhanced facilitatory processes. All responses were depressed during the onset of sleep, indicating strong inhibition. As slow-wave sleep progressed, the first and second responses increased; this was viewed as reflecting a partial release from inhibition. Disinhibition was also indicated by large increases in the fourth response. Paradoxical sleep produced still larger first and second responses, indicative of partial disinhibition.

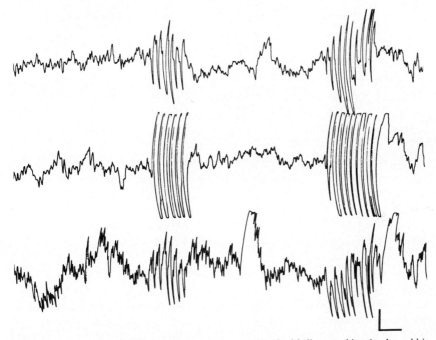

FIG. 6-15. Paroxysmal high-voltage activity associated with lip smacking in the rabbit. EEGs were obtained from 3 pairs of electrodes placed in and near the nucleus intermedius of the cerebellum. Calibrations: 20 μV; 1 sec.

2. Photic Driving as CS and US

For many years it has been known that a rhythmically flashing light evokes waves of a similar frequency over the occipital cortex. This phenomenon is known as "photic driving" and is most prominent in the EEG of man. In some human subjects, conditioned photic driving that is frequency specific can be achieved (Jus and Jus, 1960).

Studies by Morrell and Jasper (1956) employed monkeys and photic flashes of 6–12/sec as the US. During early pairings of CS and US, the CS caused generalized arousal responses followed by a driving response to the US. Later in training, an afterdischarge to flickering light appeared. Finally, conditioned repetitive responses developed. Conditioned driving was transient, however, being ultimately replaced by localized arousals in the occipital cortex only. Others have confirmed these stages of conditioning in other species.

Other studies used light flashes as the CS. In the study of dogs by Stern *et al.* (1960), light produced good EEG driving prior to establishment of a conditioned motor reflex; the driving stopped when the CR became stable. However, McAdam *et al.* (1962) found that with a CS of light flashes and a UR of leg flection photic driving increased during training in the nucleus ventralis anterior thalami and in the cortical sensory projection area.

3. Direct Brain Stimulation as CS or US

If the US of peripheral nerve stimulation is effective in conditioning, it seems reasonable to expect that a US of direct brain stimulation would be effective. Moreover, studies of this type would help indicate the brain areas involved in conditioning.

Delgado *et al.* (1954) stimulated 3 regions (midbrain, lateral thalamus, and hypothalamus) to induce fear responses. Animals were trained to turn a wheel to prevent the intracerebral shock when they heard a buzzer that preceded the shock. Conditioned responses developed readily.

High-frequency stimulation of the diffuse thalamic projection system also serves as a US which, when paired with tone as a CS, eventually leads to conditioned arousal responses in the EEG (Arias *et al.*, 1966).

Similar results were obtained by Galeano *et al.* (1964), who also studied EEG correlates. The US of electric stimulation of the midbrain reticular formation produced a fear response in cats, accompanied by EEG arousal patterns. Pairing a tone CS with the US resulted in behavioral conditioning, as well as a conditioned arousal. The EEG desynchronization in neocortex, septum, thalamus, and hypothalamus occurred early in training before behavioral CRs appeared; EEG desynchrony also persisted long after behavioral CRs had ceased during extinction trials. The CS also elicited desynchronization of olfactory bulb and amygdala activity and, in addition, caused bursts of high voltage, *fast* activity (HVFA) (Fig. 6-16). Two different arousal patterns were evident in the brain-stem reticular formation and in the dorsal hippocampus. The CS produced either theta rhythm or LVFA in the hippocampus. LVFA predominated during early trials, but when the CR was firmly established theta rhythm became dominant. Behavioral correlates included a change from LVFA to theta rhythm when the cats focused their attention on something. During extinction, some cats revealed persistent LVFA, even in the hippocampus, long after the behavioral CR and hippocampal theta activity were lost. The two aspects of reticular formation activity included the usual LVFA and a 3–5/sec slow rhythm. The classic view that reticular LVFA drives the cortex into LVFA may have some limitations, since cats sometimes showed slow reticular rhythms during cortical desynchrony.

Studies also have been performed in which brain stimulation was used as a CS. Doty *et al.* (1956) stimulated various cortical regions of cats for

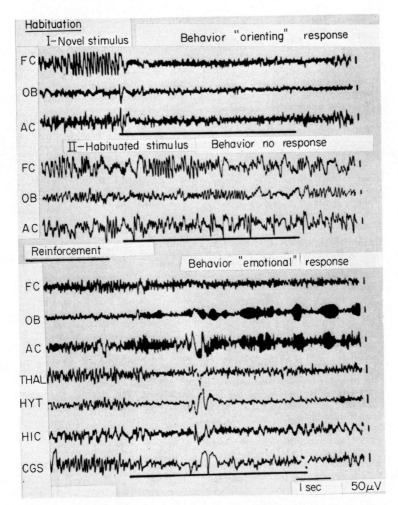

FIG. 6-16. The novel stimulus elicits a behavioral arousal (orienting) and EEG LVFA in the frontal cortex (FC), olfactory bulb (OB), and amygdala (AC) that is lost during the habituation to repeated stimulus presentations. During reinforcement with paired CS and the US, a conditioned hyperaroused state results (emotional response), associated with LVFA in most areas. Particularly noteworthy is the burst activity in the OB and AC, along with the hippocampal (HIC) LVFA instead of theta activity. Other areas monitored are the thalamus (THAL), hypothalamus (HYT), and central gray substance (CGS). (Galeano *et al.*, 1964.)

2 sec at 50 pulses/sec; if at the end of this CS, the animal still had its paw on a metal plate, the leg was shocked (US). Conditioned withdrawal responses developed readily. Circumsection of the cortical site of the CS

did not interfere with conditioning, but undercutting such areas did. Further confirmation that cortical stimulation could serve as a CS was provided in other studies in dogs, cats, and monkeys (Wells, 1963).

What can we conclude from these diverse studies? Electrographic findings suggest that no one area is responsible for conditioning. Relative emphasis given to different portions of the CNS varies with different schools of thought. Russians, wedded to Pavlovian theory, have emphasized the importance of the cerebral cortex. Western workers, dominated by ARAS theory, have tended to emphasize the role of this system. Still other workers have emphasized the hippocampus and other portions of the limbic system. All such systems are clearly involved in conditioning processes and exhibit electrographic changes indicative of their function. The memory "locus" for learned behavior is probably not to be found in any one area but rather consists of probabilistic processes operating in diffuse neural circuits, as espoused in the book by John (1967). As he puts it, "Memory is not a thing in a place but a process in a population."

C. SEDATION AND SLEEP

1. Normal Sleep

Sleep can be produced in a variety of ways. Naturally occuring sleep is a complex and still incompletely understood phenomenon. It is thought to result from the interaction of various influences: decreased alertness, fatigue, monotonous sensory input, and perhaps even chemical changes. Neurophysiologically, sleep is considered to result from deactivation of the ARAS and activation of certain inhibitory brain system, such as the diffuse thalamic projection system (DTPS) and a system in the caudal pons and rostral medulla (reviewed by Klemm, 1969).

The EEG accompaniment of sleep consists of generalized HVSA. In the cortex, especially rostral cortex, a characteristic burst pattern occurs, known as "spindling" (Fig. 6-17). Spindles are relatively high-voltage bursts of 4 or more waves with a frequency of about 6–12/sec. Under certain conditions, spindles are conspicuous in the EEG. Although the incidence, waveform, and frequency may vary slightly among species, the phenomena are considered to have similar neurophysiologic bases in all higher mammals.

In a study of spindling in unanesthetized rabbits that were gently restrained in a hammocklike sling, spindle incidence was found to vary with the state of arousal (Klemm, 1963). In the resting condition, the incidence varied from about 10 bursts/min to zero, although only a few rabbits had zero incidence. Arousing stimuli, such as saline injection or

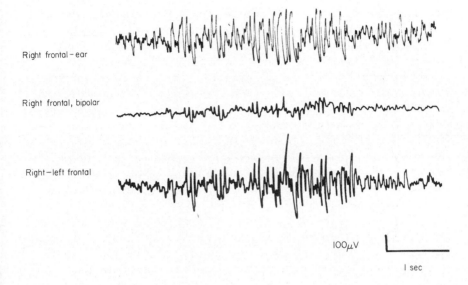

Right frontal – ear

Right frontal, bipolar

Right – left frontal

100μV

1 sec

FIG. 6-17. Illustration of spindles, as recorded from the skull of the unanesthetized rabbit. Tracings were obtained simultaneously, with 1 electrode of each pair being the same right-frontal electrode.

sham irradiation, consistently decreased spindling in those rabbits in which it was present, usually by a factor of about ⅓ for saline injection and about ½ for the sham irradiation procedure at 15 min after the stimuli were delivered. Repeated recordings on subsequent days showed that incidence was consistent within a given animal, showing very little day-to-day variation when recording conditions were kept constant.

Spindles are considered to arise from pacemaker functions of the DTPS. Alternating IPSP and EPSP changes drives the cortex in rhythmical fashion when the cortex is not dominated by tonic excitatory drive from the ARAS (Andersen and Sears, 1964).

Modern investigations of the physiology of the DTPS began with the studies of Morison and Dempsey (1942), who demonstrated the role of this system in producing the well-known recruiting phenomenon and spindles. They distinguished this system from those thalamic nuclei that specifically project afferent signals to discrete regions of the sensory cortex. Hess (1954) produced behavioral and electrographic signs of sleep by slow-frequency stimulation of this system. Later, Jasper and Drooglever-Fortuyn (1947) found that appropriate stimulation could produce the spike-wave rhythm typical of naturally occuring "petit mal" epilepsy; an arrest reaction resembling the behavioral component of petit mal also was produced (Hunter and Jasper, 1949). That same year Moruzzi and Magoun reported on the functions of the ARAS and discussed the relations of that system with the DTPS. The interrelations between the two systems is still an area of extensive investigation.

Recruiting in the rabbit is illustrated in Fig. 6-18. When the DTPS is stimulated with slow-frequency pulses (3–8/sec), predominantly negative cortical responses are evoked that grow in size (recruit) and then decline. Continuous stimulation causes a series of alternations between large and small evoked potentials. In the figure, DTPS stimulation (3 msec pulse duration, 2–6 V) produces spike and wave recruiting in the cortex and thalamus. Stimulation of the hippocampus (3 msec, pulse duration, 1.5–3 V) evokes generalized spiking in all structures. Stimulation of the ARAS (0.5 msec, 2–5 V) also induces generalized spiking. The spikes seen in the figure could be due to passive spread of stimulating current. However, it is difficult to explain why in some areas the spikes also show waxing and waning amplitudes. The best check is to study individual responses on an oscilloscope to determine spike duration (vs stimulus pulse duration) and latency of responses from the stimulus artifact. True recruiting responses develop from synaptic interactions that introduce a delay factor. Potentials similar to recruiting potentials can be evoked by slow-frequency stimulation of specific thalamic nuclei; these responses are called "augmenting" responses, and they differ from recruiting in having shorter latency and a positive phase preceding the negative wave (Buser, 1964).

Recruiting is most easily demonstrated in the sedated or sleeping animal, although it can be demonstrated in the alert animal (Evarts and Magoun, 1957; Yamaguchi et al., 1964; Fig. 6-19). Recruiting can also be evoked by low-frequency stimulation of portions of the ARAS (Lynes, 1960).

This raises the very basic consideration of relations between so-called evoked "recruiting responses" and spindling. Both the morphology and the topographical distribution of spindles and recruited waves are similar (Fig. 6-20). A close relationship between the two is also indicated by observations that spindles can be triggered by a single stimulation of the DTPS. Finally, spindles and recruited waves interact occlusively; induction of recruitment during spontaneous spindling decreases the amplitude of the spindles.

Why do spindles terminate spontaneously after a few waves, whereas recruiting can be continued much longer? Although the individual waves of a spindle result from alternating inhibitory and excitatory postsynaptic potentials, no evidence exists to explain the intervals between spindle bursts. Therefore, the following comments are very speculative.

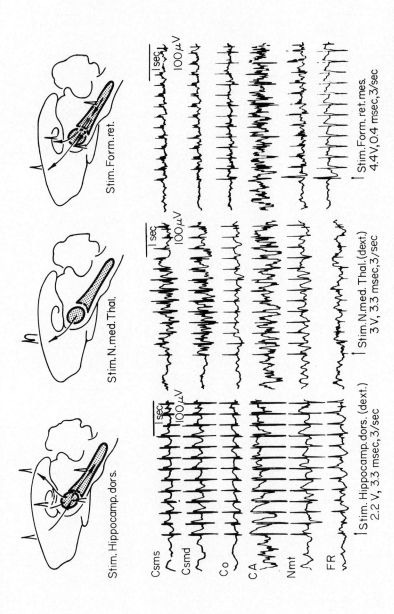

FIG. 6-18. Electrographic responses to low-frequency electric stimulation (3/sec) of dorsal hippocampus (Hippocamp. dors.), medial thalamus (N. med. Thal.), and midbrain reticular formation (Form. ret. mes.). Csms: Sensory-motor cortex; Csmd: sensory-motor cortex; Co: occipital cortex; CA: cornu ammonis (hippocampus); NmT: nucleus medial thalamus; and FR: midbrain reticular formation. (Monnier and Gangloff, 1961.)

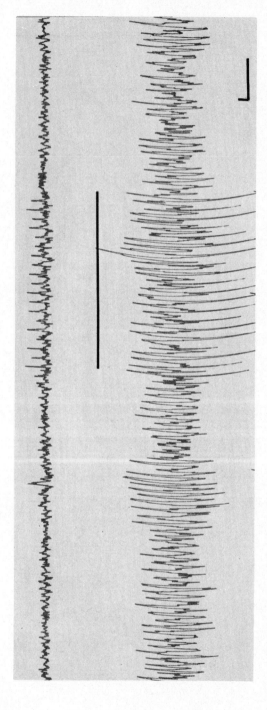

FIG. 6-19.   Recruiting responses elicited by midline thalamic stimulation (indicated by horizontal line) (0.4 msec pulses at 5/sec) in an alert rabbit (note arousal EEG pattern). Upper trace taken from the motor cortex; lower trace taken from the dorsal hippocampus. Calibration: 50 µV; 1 sec.

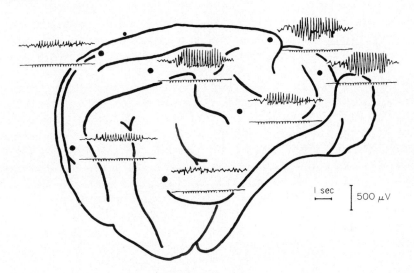

FIG. 6-20.   Recruiting response in different areas of the cerebral cortex of the cat (dial anesthesia). Stimulation of homolateral centrum medianum. (Burés *et al.*, 1967.)

Fatigue could be overridden by the artificial electric stimulation used to produce recruiting. Another consideration is that some other brain system may normally terminate a given spindle and set the delay time for the next burst; if this is done by way of inhibitory postsynaptic potentials, their time constant would be much greater than what we normally consider. Perhaps spindling initiates negative feedback through corticifugal circuits; the IPSP influence could be sustained over long periods by some sort of reverberatory network. A presynaptic inhibition mechanism could effect spindling control in a more direct fashion by being an integral part of the thalamocortical spindle circuit.

In addition to recruiting and ARAS-inhibiting functions, the DTPS is also the thalamic extension of the ARAS and can participate in behavioral and EEG arousal. Fast-frequency stimulation of the DTPS causes arousal, not recruiting (Starzl *et al.*, 1951). This effect is assumed to be indirect, acting via descending paths to the ARAS (Schlag and Chaillet, 1962).

A variety of evidence also implicates certain other brain systems that actively promote sleep, especially if animals are in a preexisting state of relaxation. Low-frequency stimulation of the caudate nucleus, cerebral cortex, hypothalamus, and various regions in the brain stem can produce sleep (reviewed by Kleitman, 1963, and Peñaloza-Rojas *et al.*, 1964). These effects may be indirect, acting through the DTPS.

A major sleep-promoting system is known to exist in the caudal pons and rostral medulla. When the pons is transected in the middle (mid-pontine, pretrigeminal preparation) and ascending influences posterior to the cut are removed, such preparations exhibit persistent cortical desynchrony (Batini *et al.*, 1958). This suggests that in the intact brain caudal brain stem structures exert a synchronizing influence, either through active inhibition of the ARAS or by triggering the DTPS. Magnes *et al.* (1961) induced cortical synchrony in intact animals by low-frequency stimulation of the solitary nucleus, pontine reticular formation, and ventral nucleus of the medulla. Favale *et al.* (1961) claim, however, that stimulation of many reticular regions in the midbrain, pons, or medulla will produce EEG synchrony and sleep; the important restrictions are that stimulation must be slower than 12/sec and that the animal must be in a preexisting relaxed state. Kumazawa (1963) claims that high-frequency stimulation (100/sec) of the ARAS will induce drowsiness, as long as the voltage is kept low.

In one study (Magora *et al.*, 1964) sleep was produced in dogs by delivery of current across the whole head. The cathode was placed over the bridge of the nose and the anode over the occiput. During the first 5 min unipolar square waves (1 msec, 100/sec) were delivered in grad-ually increasing intensity. Thereafter, the current was further increased to 7–12 mA peak and decreased in frequency to 50–20 pulses/sec.

The "hypogenic" effect of high-frequency stimulation in the Kuma-zawa and Magora studies is paradoxical inasmuch as most studies claim that only low-frequency stimulation is effective. However, Sterman and Clemente (1962) produced sleep with rapid stimulation of the pre-optic region. Also, although the relevance is not clear, Klemm (1965) en-hanced animal "hypnosis" by rapid stimulation of the pontine reticular formation.

Recently, the area postrema region of the medulla has been shown to cause EEG synchrony when it was stimulated with serotonin; Koella and Czicman (1966) present an argument that circulating serotonin activates this area, which in turn activates more rostral hypnogenic systems, causing natural sleep.

In 1957 EEG studies in man revealed that not all sleep is characterized by EEG HVSA. In fact, during a night's sleep there were transient periods of sleep when the EEG was of the arousal type. Waking and questioning the subjects at these times revealed that these were periods of dreaming.

Subsequently, similar physiologic phenomena have been observed during the sleep of many animals; in cats (Dement, 1958), chimpanzees (Adey *et al.*, 1963), birds (Klein and Jouvet, 1964), rabbits (Kawakami *et al.*, 1965), and ruminants (Jouvet and Valtax, 1962). This stage of sleep in animals has been called "rhombencephalic sleep" or "para-doxical sleep" (PS). The most comprehensive recent reviews of PS are those by Jouvet (1965) and Koella (1967).

Among the many physiologic characteristics of PS the following can be listed:

1. Arousal EEG patterns are present, with cortical LVFA and hippo-campal theta rhythms.

2. The cortical ultraslow potential shows a sudden negative shift at the beginning of PS, following the positive shift that occurs during typical sleep (Kawamura and Sawyer, 1964; Wurtz, 1965; Fig. 6-21).

3. Unit activity of certain individual neurons is increased during PS, especially in the cortex (Evarts, 1962), the ARAS (Huttenlocher, 1961), and the vestibular and geniculate nuclei (Pompeiano, 1967).

4. Nuchal EMG activity disappears.

5. Ocular movements are quite rapid and pronounced.

Some of these changes are illustrated in Fig. 6-22.

In one comparative study of sleep in birds and reptiles (Klein, 1963), the EEG of chickens and turtles changed from LFVA to HVSA as sleep ensued. Chickens, but not turtles, also exhibited episodes of LVFA during sleep, presumably PS. In a study of sleep EEGs in frogs (Hobson, 1967a,b; Fig. 6-5) neither spindles nor HVSA occurred when frogs appeared to be sleeping. Unexpectedly, frogs exhibited only LVFA during such periods, indicating that frogs do not sleep or else they only exhibit the paradoxical stage of sleep. This LVFA was not accompanied by the other usual signs of PS. The complete syndrome of PS has been reported only in young birds and mammals.

Reticular and thalamic multiple unit activity during PS in cats does not reveal the depression and burst patterns that occur during slow-wave sleep (Goodman and Mann, 1967). Rather, during PS unit activity occurs in frequent, long-duration, bursts of high amplitudes.

Mechanisms for the production of PS have been traced to systems in the brain stem, notably the pons. Ablations of the cerebral cortex or the cerebellum do not prevent electrographic indications of paradoxical sleep. Likewise, transections of the midbrain had no effect. However, transections anywhere in the anterior ⅔ of the pons DID prevent elec-trographic signs of PS (Jouvet, 1965).

Confirmation also has been obtained with localized electric stimulation studies. Stimulation of the ARAS during typical sleep (150 cps, 0.5 msec) provokes PS (Fig. 6-23). Higher intensity stimulation produces awakening rather than PS (Lissák *et al.*, 1963). Stimulation of the pontine reticular formation during typical sleep also induces PS (Jouvet, 1965).

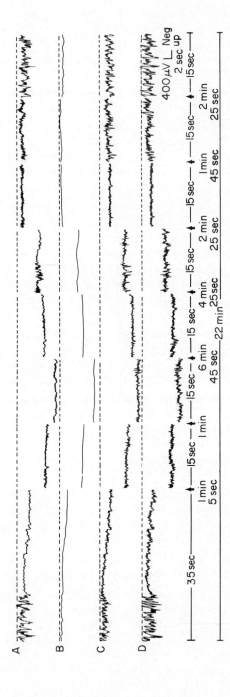

Fig. 6-21. Steady potential shifts in a cat during the transition from light sleep to wakefulness and return to light sleep. Recordings are continuous over a period of 8 min 30 sec. Arrows indicate omitted periods of record during which there were no significant changes. Recording is transcortical. A: Sigmoid gyri; B: same area, but with filtration so that frequency response is ½-amplitude at 0.5 cps; C: middle suprasylvian gyrus; and D: posterior lateral gyrus. (Wurtz, 1965.)

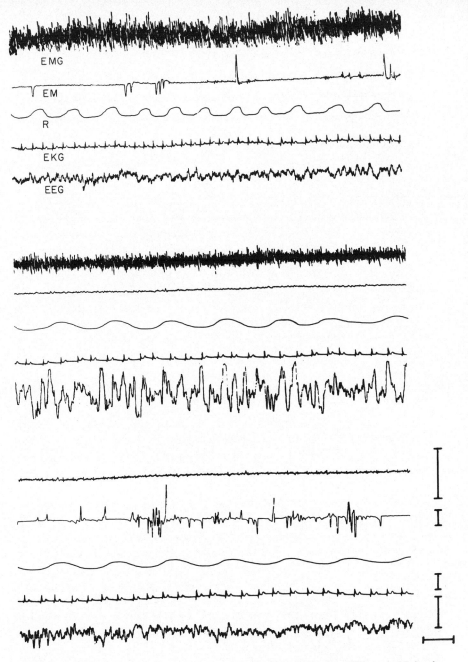

FIG. 6-22. Records illustrating physiologic changes in goats during different behavioral states. Above: Goat standing, not ruminating; middle: goat exhibiting typical sleep; and below: goat exhibiting paradoxical sleep. EMG: Electromyogram; EM: eye movement potentials; R: respiration; EKG: electrocardiogram; and EEG: frontal electroencephalogram. Calibrations: 100 μV (except 1 mV for EKG); 2 sec. (Klemm, 1966b.)

197

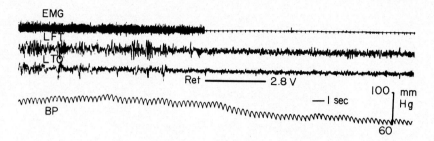

F𝐼G. 6-23. Induction of EMG, EEG [left frontal temporal (LFT) and temporal occipital cortex (LTO)] and blood pressure (BP) patterns of PS by bipolar stimulation of the midbrain reticular formation (Ret.) with 1 msec, 300/sec, and 2.8 V retangular pulses. (Modified from Candia *et al.*, 1962.)

There are several lines of evidence linking the limbic system with PS. Stimulation of the hippocampus during PS can cause a revision to the slow-wave stage of sleep (Lissák *et al.*, 1963). Also, lesions in the limbic system stop hippocampal theta rhythm, causing desynchrony; simultaneously, the number and duration of PS episodes decrease, suggesting that hippocampal theta activity helps to sustain PS (Lena and Parmeggiani, 1964).

2. *Altered Sensory Input*

The EEG can be synchronized by appropriate stimulation of cutaneous nerves. Pompeiano (1963) demonstrated this effect in freely moving cats, with the use of low-frequency stimulation of low intensity. Sometimes behavioral signs of sleep ensued. When higher intensity stimuli were used, EEG and behavioral arousal followed.

Kumazawa (1963) has described an EEG synchronizing effect of light skin pressure in the rabbit produced by application of various numbers of paper clips. More intense pressure induced EEG arousal patterns. Restraint was said to produce the same effect, unless the restraint was prolonged for about 2 hr. The inference was made that so-called animal hypnosis, a state of sustained immobility, resulted from inhibition associated with skin pressure synchronizing effects on the EEG. Hypnosis studies by the author support the concept that pressure enhances immobility, but EEG arousal patterns are much more common than relaxed patterns (Klemm, 1966a).

Distension of the carotid sinus can cause a sleeplike state in freely moving dogs and monkeys. Such distension also produces EEG sleep patterns (Bonvallet *et al.*, 1954). A more complete discussion of blood-pressure effects is found in Section III, E. Electric stimulation of vagal afferents has similar effects (Padel and Dell, 1965), presumably by activating the hypnogenic system in the caudal pons and rostral medulla that receives vagal afferents.

EEG and behavioral signs of sleep are best induced by restricting excessive sensory stimulation. Reducing the proprioceptive drive with muscle relaxants will also promote sleep (Hodes, 1961). Kleitman (1963) reviews many studies in which monotony or absence of external stimulation promote sleep in animals.

Surgical deafferentiation is a common approach to altering the influence of external stimuli. Various degrees of deafferentiation are possible, but there are 2 common preparations, both devised by Bremer (1935). In the *encéphalé isolé*, the brain is transected at the lower medulla, interrupting all sensory input except olfactory, visual, auditory, vestibular, and stimuli arising from skin and muscle of the head. Such animals exhibit a mixture of EEG signs of sleep and wakefulness. In the *cerveau isolé*, the brain is cut immediately posterior to the origin of the oculomotor nerves. All input is interrupted except for olfactory and visual stimuli. These animals exhibit only EEG sleep patterns. Batsel (1960), however, has demonstrated in *cerveau isolé* dogs that sustained episodes of arousal EEGs occasionally appeared after a week or more.

III. Internal Influences

A. OXYGEN–CARBON DIOXIDE

During the initial hypermotility and hyperpnea following ischemia of the brain, the cat EEG reveals an initial increase in frequency and amplitude. Anoxia apparently does not cause this arousal, because increased blood CO_2, in the absence of anoxia, likewise produces a transient increase in EEG frequencies. Moreover, such EEG arousals are not seen during anoxia produced by breathing oxygen-deficient air (Sugar and Gerard, 1938).

Regardless of how anoxia is produced, anoxia of moderate degree or recovery from anoxia in unanesthetized rats brings on EEG spindling and HVSA. Severe anoxia stops spindling and other EEG activity as well (Hailman *et al.*, 1943).

Restoration of oxygenation at this stage results in unusual spindle activity, in cats at least, which precedes the return of a normal EEG (Sugar and Gerard, 1938). Failure to restore oxygenation quickly leads to isoelectric EEGs and death within a few minutes.

Oxygen tensions alone do not control the reversibility of damage;

irreversible damage occurs earlier when the cause of anoxia is poor circulation than when it is due to breathing low-oxygen air (Opitz and Schneider, 1950). Ischemia, in addition to reducing oxygen supply, also produces damage through inadequate nutrient supply and waste removal. Mortality from ischemia of the brain can be reduced by hypothermia, presumably because lower temperature decrease metabolism and the dependence upon oxygen (Rosomoff, 1960).

In dogs, cardiac arrest and consequent anoxia produce a rapid onset of nearly isoelectric activity with some slow waves. If the anoxic period is short, recovery begins in a characteristic fashion, starting with low-amplitude *slow* waves that progressively increase in amplitude and frequency until normal EEGs appear (Spoerel, 1962). Duration of ischemia has been found to be logarithmically related to the latency of recovery (Brechner *et al.*, 1961).

The typical anoxic effect of HVSA has been confirmed in both dogs and cats in the studies of Gellhorn and Heymans (1948). They also noted a transient EEG arousal during recovery prior to return of normal EEGs.

Hyperoxia, generally produced by breathing high concentrations of oxygen under pressure, can be toxic. Cohn and Gersh (1945) observed in cats an initial HVSA followed by EEG seizure patterns.

Hyperventilation is a commonly used technique in human clinical EEG studies (reviewed by Brazier, 1943). Decreased blood CO_2 levels have an activating influence on many EEG abnormalities. Even in normal subjects, continued hyperventilation will induce HVSA but will not activate EEG seizures (Runnals, 1962).

In paralyzed, but unanesthetized cats, Darrow and Graf (1945) reported that 1–3 min of hyperventilation produced EEG HVSA. Direct measurements of pH of cerebrospinal fluid in anesthetized monkeys (Dusser de Barenne *et al.*, 1937) proved that hyperventilation increases pH. Small increases in pH caused increased cortical HVSA, whereas large pH increases resulted in LVFA. These workers also demonstrated the increased excitability produced by hyperventilation; the voltage required to elicit electrographic afterdischarge in monkeys was decreased. Similar demonstration of increased excitability was demonstrated by Brody and Dusser de Barenne (1932) in the motor cortex of cats.

Excessive CO_2 levels have various effects. In peripheral nerve, increased CO_2 increases stimulation threshold and conduction time (Toman, 1952). In the CNS, mild increases of CO_2 produce behavioral excitement, EEG arousal (Klemm, 1964) and excited medullary respira-

centers (Pollock, 1949). The excitement of medullary neurons may spread to the nearby ARAS and thus account for arousal responses.

Large increases in CO_2 levels produced HVSA in pigs (Mullenax and Dougherty, 1963) and isoelectric EEGs in rats (Woodbury *et al.*, 1958). The author's study of cats revealed a progression of changes in EEG as cats continued to breathe CO_2 and air: A period of HVSA and light anesthesia was followed by near isoelectric activity and deep anesthesia. These changes are in general quite similar to those that occur during more conventional types of anesthesia (Section III, F, 7). During recovery, an apparently unique EEG arousal occurred just prior to return of consciousness and persisted for many minutes after normal behavior returned. This arousal was usually confined to occipital regions, but even when found in frontal regions the LVFA always occurred first occipitally (Fig. 6-24; Klemm, 1964).

B. TEMPERATURE

Cooling of the brain can be very protective during times of stress, for example, during surgery where blood supply to the brain must be temporarily interrupted. The EEG can monitor the extent of the neural response to such cooling. Cooling of the brain of anesthetized monkeys has shown that EEG activity is abolished at about 19–22°C. Return to normal temperature restores normal EEGs, even when cooling has been extended to 9° (Bryce-Smith *et al.*, 1960).

Perfusion of the isolated heads of cats with donor blood at various temperatures revealed that EEG frequency increased as temperature rose from 20 to 38°C and decreased above that. Amplitudes also increased with increasing temperature up to about 34°, after which they decreased (Gaenshirt *et al.*, 1954).

EEGs also have been correlated in hibernating animals with body temperature and the state of hibernation. Twente and Twente (1965) found that hibernating periods were longer with lower core temperatures.

Sleep studies have indicated that brain temperatures drop slightly during slow-wave sleep but increase 0.1–0.4°C during PS (Kawamura and Sawyer, 1965).

C. CATIONS

The two most important ions affecting the EEG are potassium and calcium. Increased potassium levels usually increase EEG frequencies

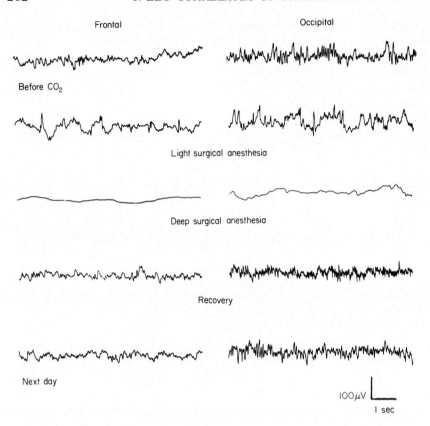

Frontal   Occipital

Before CO_2

Light surgical anesthesia

Deep surgical anesthesia

Recovery

Next day

$100 \mu V$

1 sec

FIG. 6-24. Illustration of EEG changes over frontal and occipital skull areas during and after CO_2 anesthesia in cats. Under light surgical anesthesia, high amplitude, low-frequency waves dominate; under deep surgical anesthesia, there is flattening of the waveforms, indicative of relative absence of neural function. During recovery, low amplitude, high frequencies (arousal) dominate the occipital recording. On the next day, EEGs from both areas return to normal. (Klemm, 1964.)

and neural excitability, whereas calcium, by its stabilizing effect on membrane permeability, usually has opposite effects. Dubner and Gerard (1939) demonstrated such electric activity effects in the lateral geniculate body of cats. However, Rubin et al. (1943) found that intravenous KCl or $CaCl_2$ injections had no EEG effect in anesthetized cats as long as cardiac function remained normal. Intraarterial injections would be expected to be more likely to exert an effect. Such injection of KCl to encéphalé isolé cats produced an initial, marked EEG arousal followed by HVSA. Large doses only produced initial HVSA and sometimes isoelectric activity. $CaCl_2$ injections produced HVSA that could be reversed by subsequent injections of KCl (Bonnet and Bremer, 1937).

Direct application of salts to the cortical surface produced results similar to those described for intraarterial injections (Dubner and Gerard, 1939).

Sodium injections, either intravenous or intraarterial, apparently have little effect on the EEG, as shown in studies in cats and dogs (Rubin *et al.*, 1943; Fain *et al.*, 1955). Sodium depletion, however, may have an effect. Frogs kept in distilled water exhibited low voltage, slow activity that was reversed by NaCl injection (Pick and Miller, 1945). In studies of isolated frog brain, Libet and Gerard (1939) reported that Na had an effect like K, but much greater changes in concentration were needed.

Magnesium has a marked depressant effect on brain. In isolated frog brain, Mg acted like Ca (Libet and Gerard, 1939). Although Mg can produce a fatal paralysis of skeletal respiratory muscles, anesthetic states can be produced (Smith *et al.*, 1942).

D. GLUCOSE

Glucose is the major energy source for brain functions. As such, changes in glucose levels can cause profound changes in neuronal function and the EEG.

Low blood-sugar levels, from whatever cause, initiate HVSA in the EEG. In severe hypoglycemia, isoelectric activity ensues, beginning first in the cortex; return to normal after injection of glucose occurs last in the cortex (Himwich, 1951). Such isoelectric activity has been demonstrated in unanesthetized rabbits at a time when levels were 35–50 mg/100 ml and when generalized convulsions occurred (Moruzzi, 1939).

Some conditions permit normal cortical EEGs to persist, even though glucose levels are at coma levels (Gellhorn and Kessler, 1943). Male rats in which the adrenal medullas had been removed were put into insulin coma; subsequent electric shock of the brain disrupted the coma, produced grossly normal behavior, and prompted the return of a normal EEG, although the sugar levels were still at coma level. The only explanation given for this strange phenomenon was that brain circulation must have been improved by activation of the sympathetic nervous system.

Hypoglycemia also modifies the effect of other conditions that affect the EEG. For example, hypoglycemia enhances the effect of anoxia (Gellhorn and Kessler, 1942). Low glucose also enhances the HVSA produced by hyperventilation (Hill *et al.*, 1943). In humans, hypoglycemia is known to activate latent EEG abnormalities. In one such study, of 33 patients who had normal EEGs, 17 became abnormal following tolbutamide-induced hypoglycemia (Green, 1963).

Hyperglycemia affects the EEG, tending to increase the incidence of fast frequencies. Somewhat paradoxically, injection of glucose is reported to enhance the anesthetic effect of sodium pentobarbital (Lamson *et al.*, 1951). However, in a study of dogs injection of 200 mg/kg had no apparent depressing effect on respiration or on the EEG (Hamlin *et al.*, 1965).

E. HORMONES

Thyroid hormone increases general metabolic activity, and its effect on the EEG, if any, would be expected to increase the incidence of LVFA.

Adrenal cortex hormones, especially glucocorticoids, may modify the EEG. Studies with a variety of adrenal steroids indicate that, paradoxically, some enhance excitability and seizures while others reduce irritability and raise seizure thresholds (Woodbury, 1958). Herz *et al.* (1961) reported that a single injection of ACTH caused an initial HVSA in rabbits, followed by LVFA in a few hours. There is a report that ACTH, but not hydrocortisone or desoxycorticosterone, inhibits PS; insulin has a similar effect (Kawakami *et al.*, 1966). Adrenalectomy can produce HVSA in the EEG that is reversible upon injection with glucocorticoids (Woodbury, 1958). High doses of 11-deoxy-17-hydroxycorticosterone caused an initial rhythmic high voltage, fast activity seizure in the amygdala of cats that later spread to the hippocampus and other brain areas. Following seizures, varying degrees of depression (isoelectric activity) ensued (Heuser and Eidelberg, 1961). Low doses of the same drug in monkeys produced behavioral and EEG signs of sleep, and high doses initiated seizures (Heuser *et al.*, 1965).

Single vs continuous dosage is also relevant. Low doses of 11-deoxy-17-hydroxycorticosterone given chronically raises seizure threshold, whereas a single large dose promotes seizures. Cortisol (hydrocortisone) promotes seizures when given chronically in low doses, but acute large doses have no pronounced effect (Woodbury, 1952).

Epinephrine and norepinephrine, given intravenously to adult cats, activate the EEG (Rothballer, 1956, 1959). Questions have arisen over whether this effect is direct or secondary to increased blood pressure, especially since intraventricular injections of the same agents produce somnolence (Feldberg and Sherwood, 1954).

In both avian an mammalian species, blood pressure drops during sleep (Spooner and Winters, 1966), but is this a cause or a consequence?

Epinephrine and norepinephrine have little ability to penetrate the blood–brain barrier of adult animals; this decreases the likelihood of their EEG action being direct. An indirect mechanism involving blood pressure was suggested in the studies in cats by Baust *et al.* (1963). Cortical desynchronization always occurred at or slightly later than the rise in blood pressure produced by drug injection. Mechanically induced pressure increases duplicated the drug-induced EEG activation. Destruction of the midbrain reticular formation produced HVSA that was refractory to pressure changes. Vasopressin, which also increases blood pressure, likewise induced EEG arousal patterns. Local injections of epinephrine or Ringer's solution in the midbrain reticular formation also induced alert EEG patterns, presumably from activation of pressure-sensitive neurons.

Epinephrine injection (also vasopressin and progesterone) in anesthetized rats and rabbits increased blood pressure in both species but caused EEG synchrony in rats and desynchrony in rabbits (Beyer *et al.*, 1967). These EEG changes in rats and rabbits were produced by various other means of raising blood pressure (peripheral stimulation and rapid injections of saline). Such evidence supports the idea that epinephrine effects are indirect.

The EEG synchrony in rats apparently results from increased carotid and aortic sinus discharge subsequent to pressure rise, because vasopressin had no EEG effect in denervated rats. A similar mechanism has been extensively studied in dogs, in which pressure rises also produce EEG synchrony, via sinus discharge (Bonvallet *et al.*, 1954).

However, Spooner and Winters (1967) demonstrated that many amines have direct central actions, provided they can gain access to brain tissue. They used baby chicks, which are known to have an immature blood–brain barrier that permits penetration by the amines tested. Norepinephrine and usually epinephrine induced hypertension along with EEG and behavioral signs of sleep (refer also to Kramer and Seifter, 1966). Similar EEG patterns were produced by isoproterenol and carbachol, both of which lowered blood pressure. 5-Hydroxytryptamine consistently produced depression, but pressure changes ranged from decreases to increases. Alert EEG patterns were produced by DOPA, dopamine, and amphetamine, although the pressures increased. The lack of relation between blood pressure and EEG suggests that these drug actions were direct and did not involve influences of blood pressure. These results do not necessarily exclude the possibility of pressure effects; direct actions may override vascular influences.

Sex hormonal effects on the EEG have not been widely studied. It is

known that estradiol in females increases brain excitability, as measured
by convulsive thresholds (Woolley and Timiras 1962) and by EEG
arousal thresholds (Kawakami and Sawyer, 1959). Also, rabbits display
a reaction after coitus consisting of sleep behavior and arousal EEG
patterns (now known to be PS). These reactions have been induced
spontaneously with ovulating dosages of LH gonadotropins but not
with FSH, thyrotropin, ACTH, or growth hormone (Sawyer *et al.*,
1959).

Based on reports that high doses of progesterone cause behavioral
and EEG signs of anesthesia, Heuser *et al.* (1967) studied the effects of
localized application of progesterone in the preoptic region of the
hypothalamus (known to be a sleep center). Such applications induced
long-lasting sleep with recurrent episodes of PS.

F. Pharmacologic Effects

Drugs that have been tested for their EEG effect are too numerous
for complete coverage here. An important early review was published
by Toman and Davis in 1949. Current research in this field is perhaps
most conveniently followed in *Psychopharmacological Abstracts*.[2]

1. Tranquilizers

There are many classes of tranquilizers that produce a variety of
behavior and EEG effects (Benson and Schiele, 1962). One of the best
studied classes is the phenothiazine group. These compounds generally
produce sedation as well as "tranquility." Their common EEG effects
is to produce sleep patterns with cortical spindling. Moreover, in sufficient doses, they block the typical EEG arousal response to stimuli
(Fig. 6-25). Another major group, the rauwolfia tranquilizers, is best
represented by reserpine, a drug already discussed for the EEG-behavioral dissociation it produces (Section II, A). Although the ultimate
EEG effect is one of sleep patterns, a transient alert pattern does occur.
Many of the so-called "minor tranquilizers" have little if any EEG effects.
A clinically important tranquilizer, chlordiazepoxide, is not a member
of a major group of tranquilizers but is worthy of mention because it
produces an unexpected alerting pattern after intravenous injection
(1.5–5 mg/kg) in cats; the alerting begins immediately and lasts about
4 hr, during which time the animals are tranquil but not sedated
(Roldan and Escobar, 1961).

[2]Available from the U. S. Government Printing Office.

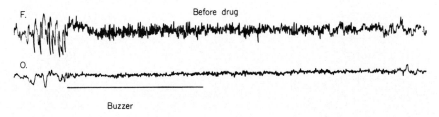

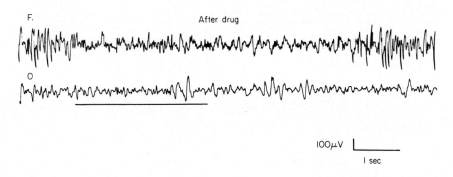

FIG. 6-25.   Illustration of chlorpromazine's blocking of the normal arousal response in both frontal (F.) and occipital (O.) areas. Note the frontal spindling before arousal and during drug influence. Records were taken with an ear reference electrode in unanesthetized rabbits. (Klemm, 1963.)

In one of the few studies on drug effects on ultraslow potential shifts, Norton and Jewett (1965a) found that chlorpromazine and amphetamine blocked potential shifts, but sedative doses of thiopental did not (Figs. 6-26a and b).

2. Antidepressants (Psychic Energizers)

Although a wide variety of compounds have clinical antidepressant effects, perhaps the best-known class of such chemicals are the monoamine oxidase inhibitors (MAOI). When given orally, these drugs require several days to develop behavioral effects that often are paralleled by emergence of persistent EEG arousal patterns (Fig. 6-27). Intravenous injections can produce EEG arousals more promptly. The MAOI, pheniprazine, produces EEG arousal when given intravenously to cats (Shimizu *et al.*, 1964). Recordings within 6 hr after intravenous injection of various MAOI drugs reveal EEG activation in rabbits (Savoldi *et al.*, 1965).

3. Acetylcholine (ACh)

ACh is a stimulant for many neurons, but intravenous injections are often not successful because of the rapid rate of enzymatic destruction. ACh effect can be demonstrated better if it is protected from enzymatic destruction by pretreatment with anticholinesterases (DFP, physostigmine, and others). Physostigmine given alone, for example, results in a generalized LVFA in cats, even when they are apparently asleep (Bradley and Elkes, 1957) or when they are sedated with the tranquilizer chlorpromazine (Bradley and Hance, 1957). Atropine reversed the ACh effect on the EEG. Neostigmine, also a cholinesterase inhibitor, apparently does not effect the EEG when given alone, even in high doses.

4. Atropine

Atropine's actions have been referred to earlier (Section II, A). It produces an apparent EEG-behavioral dissociation, wherein the EEG is of the HVSA type but behavior seems normally alert.

5. Amphetamine

Large doses (2–5 mg/kg) of amphetamine produce alert EEG patterns in conscious cats (Bradley and Elkes, 1957). At the same time behavior was changed to a more alert and excitable state. Amphetamine also greatly increased the amplitude of photically driven responses in the cortex. Similar results were noted in dogs in the study by Schallek and Walz (1953). In rabbits, amphetamine produces exaggerated theta rhythms and behavioral arousal (White and Daigneault, 1959).

6. Hallucinogens

These drugs have received much attention in recent years. Although information about such drugs is scant, it is useful to mention some reports of empirical EEG studies.

Psilocybin, in an intravenous dose of 3.5 mg/kg, produced EEG arousal patterns in the study of rabbits by Steiner and Sulman (1963). Large doses of mescaline (50 mg/kg) produced initial vomiting and arousal EEGs in cats. After about 1½ hr the cats became stuporous, and the EEGs displayed a dominant generalized 4–6/sec rhythm (Bradley and Elkes, 1957).

LSD-25, in doses of 15–25 µg/kg, produced EEG arousal changes in cats. With larger doses of 35–43 µg/kg, bursts of rhythmic 4–7/sec activity occurred that could be abolished by sensory stimulation. In encéphale isolé preparations, even massive doses produced no EEG changes, suggesting a site of action in the brain stem (Bradley and Elkes, 1957).

Intravenous injection of LSD (0.062 μmoles/kg) in rabbits caused EEG arousal reactions that were abolished by postpontine sections but not by spinal sections, suggesting a locus of action in the lower brain stem (Schweigerdt *et al.*, 1966). This agrees with the previously mentioned study in cats.

In relaxed rabbits, the large LSD dose of 0.15 mg/kg produced marked flattening of the cortical EEG, associated with absence of hippocampal theta waves. Moreover, when the reticular formation was stimulated, hippocampal theta rhythms could not be induced (Longo and Bouvet, 1964; Fig. 6-28). The LSD-induced change in hippocampal activity is difficult to explain because although the pattern is desynchronized, frequencies tended to be slower than in the relaxed, undrugged state.

Different EEGs are apparently produced in dogs. Guiti *et al.* (1966) found that oral administration of 1 μg/kg of LSD to unrestrained dogs produced a variety of behavior and increased slow frequency activity in the EEG.

The studies of rabbits by Longo and of dogs by Guiti *et al.* raise doubts about whether LSD is a "stimulant" or a "depressant"; it probably cannot be classified as either. Interesting sleep-promoting effects were reported by Hobson (1964). Within about 10 min after doses of 2 and 20 μg/kg, cats went to sleep. The EEG had a mixture of HVSA and LVFA during this sleep; often the LVFA would dominate, even though light sleep was still present. PS occurred, but it was not typical of that associated with the undrugged state. PS was manifested mainly by nuchal atonia and rapid eye movements, *without* the usual change to LVFA in the EEG. Continuous monitoring revealed that drugged cats spent less time in PS than their undrugged counterparts.

Clearly, the contradictions in the studies cited reveal our poor understanding of LSD effects on the EEG.

7. Anesthetics[3]

Barbiturates are the most common of the injectable anesthetics. They can produce, in man at least, activated EEGs just prior to the onset of unconsciousness. During the development of light pentobarbital anesthesia in cats, EEG frequencies slow to 5–7/sec and spindles become prominent over frontal areas (Clark and Ward, 1945). EEG arousal responses are difficult to produce, consisting of superposition of fast activity upon the slow rhythms and a decrease in slow-rhythm amplitude. At surgical levels of anesthesia, the EEG is generally considered completely unresponsive to arousal stimuli. However, Prince and

---

[3]For a more complete neurophysiologic review, refer to Winters *et al.* (1967).

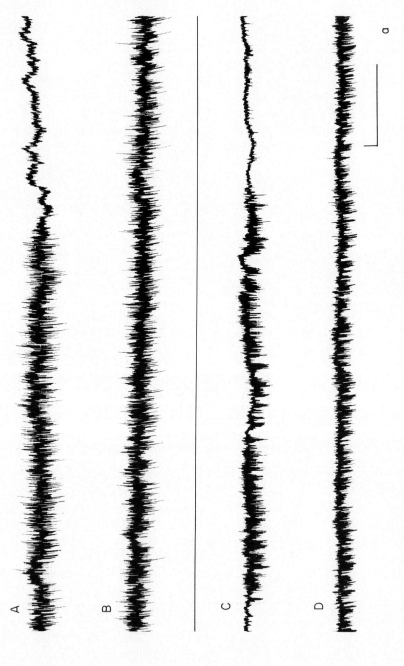

Fig. 6-26. (a) Effect of chlorpromazine on EEG slow potentials. A: Records from a control cat during slow-wave sleep and PS, both showing the same potentials; B: records from same cat ½ hr after chlorpromazine (2 mg/kg), illustrating blockage of PS and a depression of the slow waves; C: control recordings from another cat illustrating light sleep and PS, both accompanied by 0.7/min waves; and D: records from

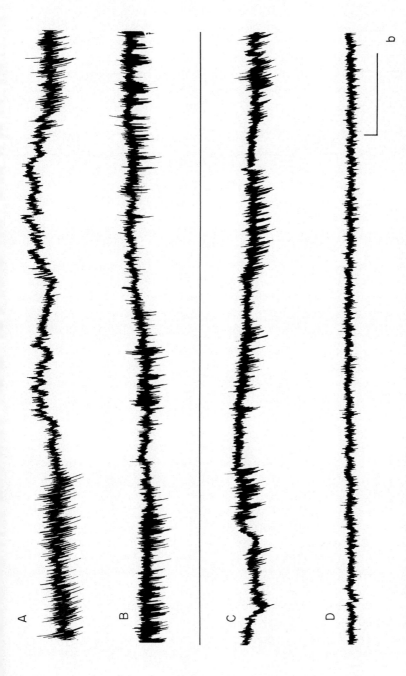

Fig. 6-26. (b) Effect of amphetamine of EEG slow potentials. A: Control record showing light sleep and PS; B: same cat ½ hr after amphetamine (0.25 mg/kg), showing slight depression of large oscillations; C: another cat control record during light sleep with 1/min oscillations; and D: records from same cat 1 hr after amphetamine (1 mg/kg), showing no major oscillations, although slow waves of 11/min are present. Calibrations: 200 μV; 1 min, negative up. (Norton and Jewett, 1965a.)

Shanzer (1966) report that arousing stimuli can induce a paradoxical cortical HVSA in anesthetized cats. In very deep anesthesia, isoelectric periods ensue from which emerge bursts of slow monophasic spindles or isolated sharp waves (so-called "burst suppression"). At still deeper levels of anesthesia, the EEG becomes completely isoelectric; activity returns as the anesthetic is metabolized. These changes are similar to those described by Drohocki and Drohocka (1939) after their study of several species of animals.

Subcortical electric activity in normal, anesthetized cats has been described by Brooks (1962). Of special interest is the report of pronounced spiking that occurs normally in the hippocampus, ventromedial hypothalamic nucleus, and prepyriform cortex at deeper levels of anesthesia. In very deep anesthesia, these spikes appear in neocortex. Clearly, such discharges should not be interpreted to indicate disease.

The HVSA that appears during surgical anesthesia does contain truly periodic components, shown by autocorrelation to be about 5–6/sec in cats (Brazier, 1963). Similar findings were noted when the HVSA was caused by other anesthetics or even by natural sleep. Since such periodicity is conspicuously absent or limited in alert cats, and probably other nonhuman animals, sleep or depressant drugs may remove an inhibitory influence and thus uncover a normally suppressed rhythm.

Studies to provide clinical control data in anesthetized dogs (Klemm, 1968) revealed that the EEG is very stable during light anesthesia induced by sodium pentobarbital. Interval histogram data comparing wave durations at one time with those 30 min later from the same dog are shown in Fig. 6-29. Although up to 2-fold differences among dogs in EEG amplitudes occurred, the wave durations were reasonably consistent. The basic EEG waves (small, superimposed activity was removed by filtration) revealed presence of a broad spectrum of frequencies (refer to Fig. 5-10). Spindles were most conspicuous in recordings with a reference electrode; the incidence ranged from 4 to 9 bursts/min. Spindles were of 2 basic types: one a relatively high-amplitude form and the other a masked form in which spindles consisted of a superimposed low-voltage ripple. Deep anesthesia (Plane 3, Guedel scheme) produced EEGs similar to those during light anesthesia, except that some mild slowing was evident. In some animals, deep anesthesia abolished spindling, although when it was present characteristics were similar to that noted during light anesthesia. In still deeper planes of anesthesia, "burst suppression" was observed (Fig. 6-30).

Barbiturates have interesting actions on evoked responses that are enlightening on the qualities of "anesthesia." The highly localized, brief,

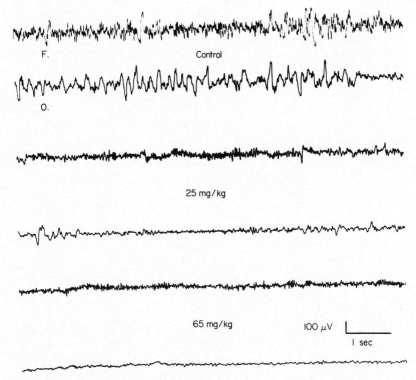

FIG. 6-27.   Records illustrating the EEG activation produced by the MAOI nialamide. When given 3 daily doses of 25 mg/kg, the EEG in both frontal (F.) and occipital (O.) areas accelerated greatly. When a dose of 65 mg/kg was administered, the increase was still more noticeable. Records taken with an ear reference in unanesthetized rabbits. (Klemm, 1963.)

monophasic surface positive cortical responses that occur from specific afferent input are not greatly depressed by anesthesia. The major effect on primary responses is one of increasing the recovery time (Marshall *et al.*, 1941; Bureš *et al.*, 1967). These findings suggest that primary sensory information is received at the cortex; anesthesia therefore must act mainly on the processing of sensory information. Support for such a concept comes from analyses of late components in cortical evoked responses. Latency and diffuseness of secondary evoked responses vary with the degree of central synaptic processing of primary sensory input. Marshall *et al.* (1941) reported anesthetic depression of later components in the evoked response. Similarly, Forbes and Morison (1939) observed little anesthetic effect on the localized primary responses but considerable depression of the later and more diffuse secondary responses.

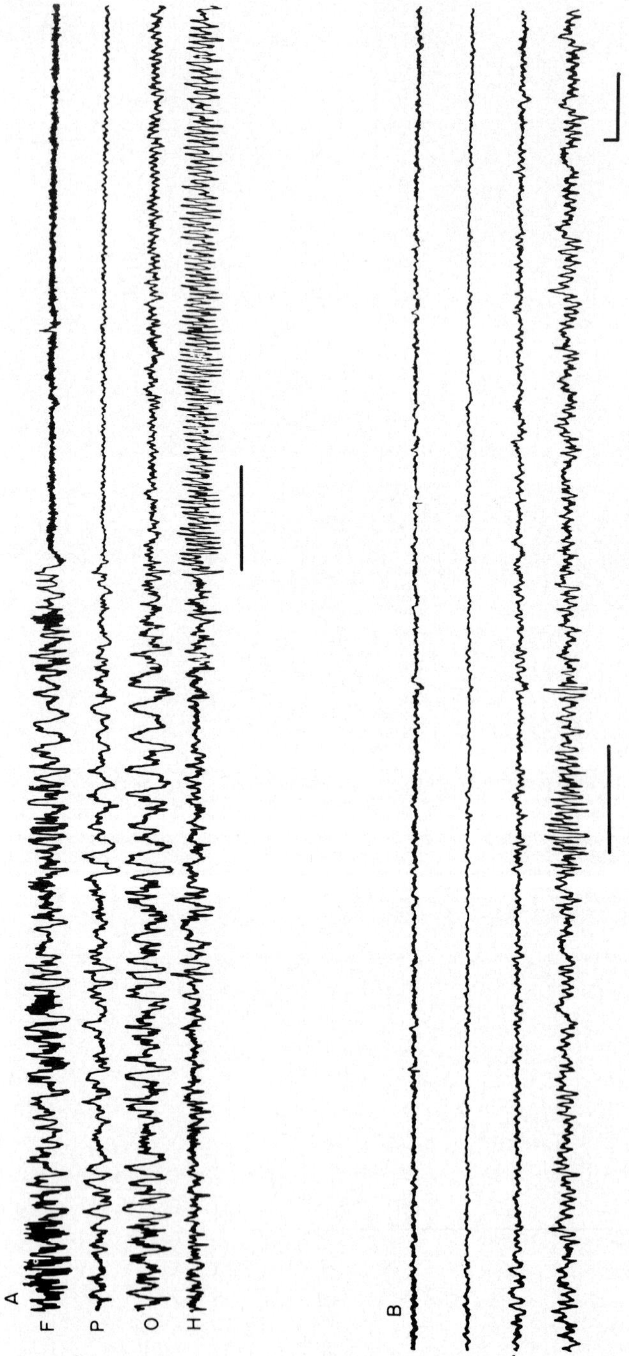

Fig. 6-28.　A: EEG activation produced by electric stimulation of the reticular formation; B: after 0.15 mg/kg LSD, the tracing is flattened, and hippocampal theta waves are no longer observed after reticular stimulation. At the horizontal line: stimulation of reticular formation, 0.4 V, 250 cps, and 0.1 msec pulses. F: Left posterior sensorimotor cortex; P: left anterior sensorimotor cortex; O: left optic cortex; and H: left dorsal hippocampus. Calibrations: 100 μV; 2 sec. (Longo and Bouvet, 1964.)

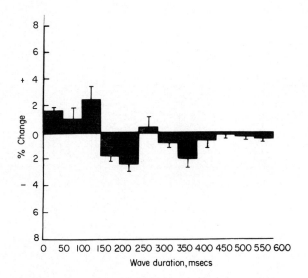

FIG. 6-29. Stability of the EEG with time in lightly anesthetized dogs. Interval histogram data are averages from a bipolar arrangement on 5 dogs. Paired comparison is made
between the distribution at one time with that 30 min later. Deviations shown = 1 SE.
(Klemm, 1968.)

Important experiments by French and King (1955) revealed that pain-
induced impulses in spinothalamic pathways were generally unimpaired
by anesthesia during propagation to the sensory cortex, whereas the
responses evoked in the ARAS were greatly depressed. Depression of
sensory collateral impulses in the ARAS is interpreted to mean that the
information contained in primary sensory paths is not "processed."
Bases thus are laid for saying that sensory information during anesthesia
is "received" but not "perceived."

Ether anesthesia in the dog produces an initial amplitude increase
in fast (50/sec) components. In deep anesthesia, *low*-voltage slow waves
dominate the record. Spindles become evident during recovery (Swank
and Watson, 1949). In cats, ether produces mixtures of fast and slow
activity during light anesthesia and HVSA during deep anesthesia
(Forbes *et al.*, 1935). Rabbits display a marked EEG arousal reaction
during induction with ether. This activity persists, mixed with low-
voltage slow activity during anesthesia (Bureš *et al.*, 1967). Other differences between ether and barbiturates and the effects of other anesthetics are summarized by Toman and Davis (1949) and Root and
Hofmann (1963).

Individual neuronal discharge in many brain regions is suppressed by
anesthesia, even at a time when EEG signals are still recordable (Chap-

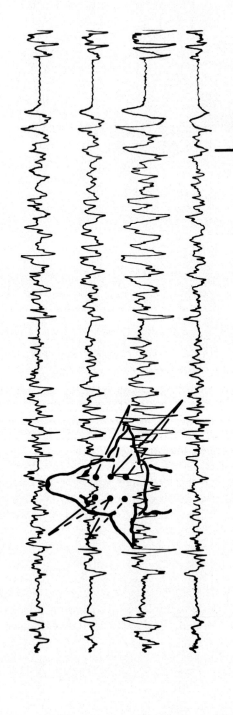

FIG. 6-30. "Burst suppression" or periods of relative electric silence during deep anesthesia in the dog. Calibrations: 20 μV; 1 sec. (Klemm, 1968.)

ter 1). Reticular and thalamic multiple unit activity in cats tends to be differentially influenced by various anesthetics, but in all instances activity decreases and occurs in bursts, similar to the observations during slow-wave sleep (Goodman and Mann, 1967).

Ultraslow potentials shift during anesthesia, with a polarity that is opposite that produced during alert wakefulness or after administration of arousal-producing drugs (reviewed by Norton and Jewett, 1965a).

REFERENCES

Adey, W. R., Dunlop, C. W., and Hendrix, C. E. (1960). Hippocampal slow waves. Distribution and phase relationships in the course of approach learning. *Arch. Neurol.* **3**, 74–90.

Adey, W. R., Kado, R. T., and Rhodes, J. M. (1963). Sleep: Cortical and subcortical recordings in the chimpanzee. *Science* **141**, 923–933.

Ajmone Marsan, C. (1965). Micro-structural mechanisms of seizure susceptibility. *Excerpta Med. Found., Intern. Congr. Ser.* **124**, 47–59.

Andersen, P., and Sears, T. A. (1964). The role of inhibition in the phasing of spontaneous thalamo—cortical discharge. *J. Physiol. (London)* **173**, 459–480.

Arias, L. P., Ross, N., and Piñeyrua, M. (1966). Stimulation of the nonspecific thalamic nuclei in relation to conditioning. *Exptl. Neurol.* **16**, 93–103.

Batini, C., Moruzzi, G., Palestini, M., Rossi, G. F., and Zanchetti, A. (1958). Persistent patterns of wakefulness in the pretrigeminal midpontine preparation. *Science* **128**, 30–32.

Batsel, H. L. (1960). Electroencephalographic synchronization and desynchronization in the chronic "cerveau isolé" of the dog. *Electroencephalog. Clin. Neurophysiol.* **12**, 421–430.

Baust, W., Niemczyk, H., and Vieth, J. (1963). The action of blood pressure on the ascending reticular activating system with special reference to adrenaline-induced arousal. *Electroencephalog. Clin. Neurophysiol.* **15**, 63–72.

Beck, E. C., Doty, R. W., and Kooi, K. A. (1958). Electrocortical reactions associated with conditioned flexion reflexes. *Electroencephalog. Clin. Neurophysiol.* **10**, 279–289.

Benson, W. M., and Schiele, B. C. (1962). "Tranquilizing and Anti-Depressive Drugs." Thomas, Springfield, Illinois.

Beyer, C., Ramirez, V. D., Whitmoyer, D. I., and Sawyer, C. H. (1967). Effects of hormones on the electrical activity of the brain in the rat and rabbit. *Exptl. Neurol.* **18**, 313–326.

Bonnet, V., and Bremer, F. (1937). Action du potassium, du calcium et de l'acétylcholine sur les activitiés electriques, spontanées et provoquées, de l'écoree cérébrale. *Compt. Rend. Soc. Biol.* **126**, 1271–1275.

Bonvallet, M., Dell, P., and Hiebel, G. (1954). Tonus sympathique et activité électrique corticale. *Electroencephalog. Clin. Neurophysiol.* **6**, 119–144.

Bradley, P. B., and Elkes, J. (1957). The effects of some drugs on the electrical activity of the brain. *Brain* **80**, 77–117.

Bradley, P. B., and Hance, A. J. (1957). The effect of chlorpromazine and methopromazine on the electrical activity of the brain of the cat. *Electroencephalog. Clin. Neurophysiol.* **9**, 191–215.

Brazier, M. A. B. (1943). The physiological effects of carbon dioxide on the activity of the central nervous system in man. *Medicine* **22**, 205–221.

Brazier, M. A. B. (1963). The problem of periodicity in the electroencephalogram: Studies in the cat. *Electroencephalog. Clin. Neurophysiol.* **15**, 287–298.

Brechner, V. L., Bethune, R. W. M., Kavan, E. M., Bauer, R. O., Phillips, R. E., and Dillon, J. B. (1961). The encephalographic effect of arrested circulation in the normothermic human and dog. *Anesthesia Analgesia, Current Res.* **40**, 1–14.

Bremer, F. (1935). Cerveau "isolé" et physiologie du sommeil. *Compt. Rend Soc. Biol.* **118**, 1235–1241.

Brody, B. S., and Dusser de Barenne, J. G. (1932). Effect of hyperventilation on the excitability of the motor cortex in cats. *A.M.A. Arch. Neurol. Psychiat.* **28**, 571–585.

Brooks, D. C. (1962). Rhinencephalic spikes and beta waves in the cat under pentobarbital. *Am. J. Physiol.* **202**, 1221–1229.

Bryce-Smith, R., Epstein, H. G., and Glees, P. (1960). Physiological studies during hypothermia in monkeys. *J. Appl. Physiol.* **15**, 440–444.

Buchwald, J. S., Halas, E. S., and Schramm, S. (1966). Relationships of neuronal spike populations and EEG activity in chronic cats. *Electroencephalog. Clin. Neurophysiol.* **21**, 227–238.

Bureš, J., Petráň, M., and Zachar, J., eds. (1967). "Electrophysiological Methods in Biological Research," 3rd rev. ed. Academic Press, New York.

Buser, P. (1964). Thalamic influences on the EEG. *Electronencephalog Clin. Neurophysiol.* **16**, 18–26.

Candia, O., Favale, E., Giussani, A., and Rossi, G. F. (1962). Blood pressure during natural sleep and during sleep induced by electrical stimulation of the brain stem reticular formation. *Arch. Ital. Biol.* **100**, 216–233.

Caspers, H. (1961). Changes of cortical D.C. potentials in the sleep-wakefulness cycle. Ciba Found. Symp., *The Nature of Sleep*, pp. 237–253.

Chertok, L., and Kramarz, P. (1959). Hypnosis, sleep, and electroencephalography. *J. Nervous Mental Disease* **128**, 227–238.

Clark, S. L., and Ward, J. W. (1945). Electroencephalogram of different cortical regions of normal and anesthetized cats. *J. Neurophysiol.* **8**, 99–112.

Cohn, R., and Gersh, I. (1945). Changes in brain potentials during convulsions induced by oxygen under pressure. *J. Neurophysiol.* **8**, 155–160.

Darrow, C. W., and Graf, C. G. (1945). Relation of electroencephalogram and psychophysiological regulation in the brain. *Am. J. Psychiat.* **102**, 791–798.

Delgado, J. M. R., Roberts, W. W., and Miller, N. E. (1954). Learning motivated by electrical stimulation of the brain. *Am. J. Physiol.* **179**, 587–593.

Dement, W. (1958). The occurrence of low voltage, fast, electroencephalogram patterns during behavioral sleep in the cat. *Electroencephalog. Clin. Neurophysiol.* **10**, 291–296.

Demetrescu, M., Demetrescu, M., and Iosif, G. (1966). Diffuse regulation of visual thalamocortical responsiveness during sleep and wakefulness. *Electroencephalog. Clin. Neurophysiol.* **20**, 450–469.

Doty, R. W., Rutledge, L. T., and Larsen, R. M. (1956). Conditioned reflexes established to electrical stimulation of cat cerebral cortex. *J. Neurophysiol.* **19**, 401–415.

Drohocki, Z., and Drohocka, J. (1939). Etudé électroencéphalographique de la localisation pharmacologique des narcotiques. *Arch. Intern. Pharmacodyn.* **62**, 265–279.

Dubner, H. H., and Gerard, R. W. (1939). Factors controlling brain potentials in the cat. *J. Neurophysiol.* **2**, 142–152.

Dusser de Barenne, J. G., McCulloch, W. S., and Nims, L. F. (1937). Functional activity and pH of the cerebral cortex. *J. Cellular Comp. Physiol.* **10**, 277–289.

Eccles, J. C. (1964). "The Physiology of Synapses." Springer, Berlin.

Evarts, E. V. (1962). Activity of neurons in visual cortex of the cat during sleep with low voltage fast activity. *J. Neurophysiol.* **25**, 812–816.

Evarts, E. V., and Magoun, H. W. (1957). Some characteristics of cortical recruiting responses in unanesthetized cats. *Science* **125**, 1147–1148.

Fain, P., Dennis, J., and Harbaugh, F. B. (1955). Influence of potassium ions on the electroencephalogram of the dog. *Am. J. Physiol.* **182**, 415-418.

Favale, E., Loeb, C., Rossi, G. F., and Sacco, G. (1961). EEG synchronization and behavioral signs of sleep following low frequency stimulation of the brain stem reticular formation. *Arch. Ital. Biol.* **99**, 1-22.

Feldberg, W., and Sherwood, S. L. (1954). Injections of drugs into the lateral ventricle of the cat. *J. Physiol. (London)* **123**, 148-167.

Flexner, L. B., Tyler, D. B., and Gallant, L. J. (1950). Biochemical and physiological differentiation during morphogenesis. *J. Neurophysiol.* **13**, 427-430.

Forbes, A., and Morison, B. R. (1939). Cortical response to sensory stimulation under deep barbiturate narcosis. *J. Neurophysiol.* **2**, 112-128.

Forbes, A., Derbyshire, A. J., Rempel, B., and Lambert, E. (1935). The effects of ether, nembutal, and avertin on the potential patterns of the motor cortex. *Am. J. Physiol.* **113**, 43-44.

Fox, M. W. (1964). Effects of pentobarbital on the EEG of maturing dogs and a review of the literature. *Vet. Record* **76**, 768-770.

Fox, M. W. (1967). Postnatal development of the EEG in the dog. Parts I, II, and III. *J. Small Animal Pract.* **8**, 71-112.

French, J. D., and King, E. E. (1955). Mechanisms involved in the anesthetic state. *Surgery* **38**, 228-238.

Gaenshirt, H., Krenkel, W., and Zylka, W. (1954). The electrocorticogram of the cat's brain at temperatures between 40°C and 20°C. *Electroencephalog. Clin. Neurophysiol.* **6**, 409-413.

Galeano, C., Prieto, S., Ross, N., Piñeyrua, M., Stirner, A., and Arias, L. P. (1964). *Acta Neurol. Latinoam.* **10**, 137-152.

Gellhorn, E., and Heymans, C. (1948). Differential action of anoxia, asphyxia and carbon dioxide on normal and convulsive potentials. *J. Neurophysiol.* **11**, 261-273.

Gellhorn, E., and Kessler, M. (1942). The effect of hypoglycemia on the electroencephalogram at varying degrees of oxygenation of the blood. *Am. J. Physiol.* **136**, 1-6.

Gellhorn, E., and Kessler, M. (1943). Interaction of electric shock and insulin hypoglycemia. *A.M.A. Arch Neurol. Psychiat.* **49**, 808-819.

Goodman, S. J., and Mann, P. E. G. (1967). Reticular and thalamic multiple unit activity during wakefulness, sleep and anesthesia. *Exptl. Neurol.* **19**, 11-24.

Grástyan, E., Lissák, K., Madarasz, I., and Donhoffer, H. (1959). Hippocampal electrical activity during the development of conditioned reflexes. *Electroencephalog. Clin. Neurophysiol.* **11**, 409-430.

Green, J. B. (1963). The activation of electroencephalographic abnormalities by tolbutamide-induced hypoglycemia. *Neurology* **13**, 192-200.

Green, J. D., and Arduini, A. A. (1954). Hippocampal electrical activity in arousal. *J. Neurophysiol.* **17**, 533-557.

Grossman, C. (1955). Electro-ontogenesis of cerebral activity. *A.M.A. Arch. Neurol. Psychiat.* **74**, 186-202.

Guiti, N., Djahanguiri, B., and Mehdizadeh, H. (1966). Analyse quantitative d'électro-encéphalogrammes répétés chez le chien soumis a l'effet du diéthyl lysergamide (LDS$_{25}$). *Electroencephalog. Clin. Neurophysiol.* **21**, 80-84.

Hailman, H., Kessler, M., and Gellhorn, E. (1943). Influence of lowered barometric pressure on the electroencephalogram. *Proc. Soc. Exptl. Biol. Med.* **54**, 74-76.

Hamlin, R. L., Redding, R. W., Rieger, J. E., Smith, R. C., and Prynn, R. B. (1965). Insignificance of the "glucose effect" in dogs anesthetized with pentobarbital. *J. Am. Vet. Med. Assoc.* **146**, 238-241.

Hayward, J. N., Fairchild, M. D., and Stuart, D. G. (1966). Hypothalamic and cortical D-C potential changes induced by stimulation of the midbrain reticular formation. *Exptl. Brain Res.* 1, 205–219.

Heim, L. (1967). Brain maturation in the neonatal rat after varied light cycles. *Proc. Soc. Exptl. Biol. Med.* 124, 223–225.

Herz, A., Krupp, P., and Monnier, M. (1961). Uber die Wirkung von ACTH und Steroid-hormonen auf die elektrische Aktivität des Gehirns. *Arch. Ges. Physiol.* 272, 442–462.

Hess, W. R. (1954). The diencephalic sleep centre. *In* "Brain Mechanisms and Consciousness" (J. F. Delafresnaye, ed.), pp. 117–136. Blackwell, Oxford.

Heuser, G., and Eidelberg, E. (1961). Steroid-induced convulsions in experimental animals. *Endocrinology* 69, 915–924.

Heuser, G., Ling, G. M., and Buchwald, N. A. (1965). Sedation or seizures as dose-dependent effects of steroids. *Arch. Neurol. Psychiat.* 13, 195–203.

Heuser, G., Ling, G. M., and Kluver, M. (1967). Sleep induction by progesterone in the pre-optic area in cats. *Electroencephalog. Clin. Neurophysiol.* 22, 122–127.

Hill, D., Sargant, W., and Heppenstall, M. E. (1943). A case of matricide. *Lancet* 1, 526–527.

Himwich, H. E. (1951). "Brain Metabolism and Cerebral Disorders." Williams & Wilkins, Baltimore, Maryland.

Hobson, J. A. (1964). The effect of LSD on the sleep cycle of the cat. *Electroencephalog. Clin. Neurophysiol.* 17, 52–56.

Hobson, J. A. (1967a). Electrographic correlates of behavior in the frog with special reference to sleep. *Electroencephalog. Clin. Neurophysiol.* 22, 113–121.

Hobson, J. A. (1967b). Respiration and EEG synchronization in the frog. *Nature* 213, 988–989.

Hodes, R. (1961). Electrocortical synchronization (EGS) in cats from reduction of proprioceptive drive caused by a muscle relaxant (Flaxedil). *Federation Proc.* 20, 332 (Abstract).

Hunter, J., and Jasper, H. H. (1949). Effects of thalamic stimulation in unanesthetized animals; arrest reaction and petit mal seizures, activation patterns and generalized convulsions. *Electroencephalog. Clin. Neurophysiol.* 1, 305–324.

Huttenlocher, P. R. (1961). Evoked and spontaneous activity in single units of medial brain stem during natural sleep and waking. *J. Neurophysiol.* 24, 451–468.

Jasper, H. H., and Droogleever-Fortuyn, J. (1947). Experimental studies on the functional anatomy of petit mal epilepsy. *Res. Publ., Assoc. Res. Nervous Mental Disease* 26, 272–298.

Jasper, H. H., Bridgman, C. S., and Carmichael, L. (1937). Ontogenic study of cerebral electrical potentials in guinea-pig. *J. Exptl. Psychol.* 21, 63–71.

John, E. R. (1967). "Mechanisms of Memory." Academic Press, New York.

Jouvet, D., and Valtax, J. L. (1962). Etude polygraphique du sommeil chez l'agneau. *Compt. Rend. Soc. Biol.* 156, 1411–1414.

Jouvet, M. (1965). Paradoxical sleep — A study of its nature and mechanisms. *Prog. Brain Res.* 18, 20–62.

Jus, A., and Jus, C. (1960). Étude de l'extinction par répétition de l'expression EEG du réflexe d'orientation et de l'action du frein externe sur les réactions EEG aux différents stimuli chez l'homme. *Electroencephalog. Clin. Neurophysiol.* Suppl. 13, 321–333.

Kawakami, M., and Sawyer, C. H. (1959). Changes in brain activity thresholds by sex steroids. *Endocrinology* 65, 652 (refer also to Sawyer *et al.*, 1959).

Kawakami, M., and Sawyer, C. H. (1959). Changes in brain activity thresholds by sex steroids. *Endocrinology* 65, 652 (refer also to Sawyer *et al.*, 1959).

Kawakami, M., Negoro, H., and Takahashi, T. (1966). Neuropharmacological studies on the mechanisms of paradoxical sleep in the rabbit. *Japan. J. Physiol.* 16, 667–683.

Kawamura, H., and Sawyer, C. H. (1964). D-C potential changes in rabbit brain during slow-wave and paradoxical sleep. *Am. J. Physiol.* **207**, 1379–1386.

Kawamura, H., and Sawyer, C. H. (1965). Elevation in brain temperature during paradoxical sleep. *Science* **150**, 912–913.

Kennard, M. A., and Nims, L. F. (1942). Changes in normal EEG of Macaca Mulatta with growth. *J. Neurophysiol.* **5**, 325–333.

Klein, M. (1963). "Étude polygraphique et phylogénique des états de sommeil." Bosc, Lyon.

Klein, M., Michel, F., and Jouvet, M. (1964). Étude polygraphique du sommeil chez les oiseaux. *Compt. Rend. Soc. Biol.* **158**, 99–103.

Kleitman, N. (1963). "Sleep and Wakefulness." Univ. of Chicago Press, Chicago, Illinois.

Klemm, W. R. (1963). Protection against x-irradiation by psychotropic drugs and adrenal-pituitary function on rabbit behavior and brain electrical activity. Ph.D. thesis, University of Notre Dame, Notre Dame, Indiana.

Klemm, W. R. (1964). Carbon dioxide anesthesia in cats. *Am. J. Vet. Res.* **25**, 1201–1205.

Klemm, W. R. (1965). Potentiation of animal "hypnosis" with low-level electric current stimulation. *Animal Behav.* **13**, 571–574.

Klemm, W. R. (1966a). Electroencephalographic-behavioral dissociations during animal hypnosis. *Electroencephalog. Clin. Neurophysiol.* **21**, 365–372.

Klemm, W. R. (1966b). Sleep and paradoxical sleep in ruminants. *Proc. Soc. Exptl. Biol. Med.* **121**, 635–638.

Klemm, W. R. (1968). Subjective and quantitative analyses of the electroencephalogram of anesthetized normal dogs: Control data for clinical diagnosis. *Am. J. Vet. Res.* **29**, 1267–1277.

Klemm, W. R. (1969). Sleep and wakefulness. *In* "Dukes' Physiology of Domestic Animals" (M. J. Swenson, ed.). Cornell Univ. Press, Ithaca, New York (in press).

Koella, W. P. (1967). "Sleep." Thomas, Springfield, Illinois.

Koella, W. P., and Czicman, J. (1966). Mechanism of the EEG synchronizing action of serotonin. *Am. J. Physiol.* **211**, 926–934.

Kramer, S. Z., and Seifter, J. (1966). The effects of gaba and biogenic amines on behavior and brain electrical activity in chicks. *Life Sci.* **5**, 527–534.

Kumazawa, T. (1963). "Deactivation" of the rabbit's brain by pressure application to the skin. *Electroencephalog. Clin. Neurophysiol.* **15**, 660–671.

Lamson, P. D., Greig, M. G., and Hobdy, C. J. (1951). Modification of barbiturate anesthesia by glucose intermediary metabolites and certain other substances. *J. Pharmaco. Exptl. Therap.* **103**, 460–470.

Lena, C., and Parmeggiani, P. L. (1964). Hippocampal theta rhythm and activated sleep. *Helv. Physiol. Pharmacol. Acta* **22**, 120–135.

Libet, B., and Gerard, R. W. (1939). Control of the potential rhythm of the isolated frog brain. *J. Neurophysiol.* **2**, 153–169.

Lindsley, D. B. (1952). Psychological phenomena and the electroencephalogram. *Electroencephalog. Clin. Neurophysiol.* **4**, 443–456.

Lissák, K., Karmos, G., and Grastyán, E. (1963). A study of the so-called "paradoxical" phase of sleep in cats. *Prog. Brain Res.* **1**, 424–428.

Longo, V. G. (1966). Behavioral and electroencephalographic effects of atropine and related compounds. *Pharmacol. Rev.* **18**, 965–996.

Longo, V. G., and Bouvet, D. (1964). A neuropharmacological investigation on hallucinogenic drugs. Laboratory results versus clinical trials. *Acta Neurochir.* **12**, 215–229.

Loomis, A. L., Harvey, E. N., and Hobart, G. (1936). Brain potentials during hypnosis. *Science* **83**, 239–241.

Lynes, T. E. (1960). A cortical recruiting response elicited by low frequency stimulation of the mesencephalic reticular formation. *Federation Proc.* **19**, 293.

McAdam, D. W., Knott, J. R., and Ingram, W. R. (1962). Changes in EEG responses evoked by the conditioned stimulus during classical aversive conditioning in the cat. *Electroencephalog. Clin. Neurophysiol.* **14**, 731–738.

Magnes, J., Moruzzi, G., and Pompeiano, O. (1961). Synchronization of the EEG by low-frequency electrical stimulation of the region of the solitary tract. *Arch. Ital. Biol.* **99**, 33–67.

Magora, F., Beller, A., and Aladjemoff, L. (1964). Electrical sleep in dogs. *Brit. J. Anaesthesia* **36**, 407–414.

Marshall, W. H., Woolsey, C. N., and Bard, P. (1941). Observations on cortical somatic sensory mechanisms of cat and monkey. *J. Neurophysiol.* **4**, 1–24.

Monnier, M., and Gangloff, H. (1961). "Atlas for Stereotaxic Brain Research on the Conscious Rabbit." Elsevier, Amsterdam.

Morison, R. S., and Dempsey, E. W. (1942). A study of thalamo-cortical relations. *Am. J. Physiol.* **135**, 281–292.

Morrell, F., and Jasper, H. H. (1956). Electrographic studies of the formation of temporary connections in the brain. *Electroencephalog. Clin. Neurophysiol.* **8**, 201–215.

Moruzzi, G. (1939). Étude de l'activité électrique de l'écorce cérébrale dans l'hypoglucémie insulinque et dans différentes conditions modifiant le métabolisme des centres. *Arch. Intern. Physiol.* **48**, 45–101.

Moruzzi, G., and Magoun, H. W. (1949). Brain-stem reticular formation and activation of the EEG. *Electroencephalog. Clin. Neurophysiol.* **1**, 455–473.

Mullenax, C. H., and Dougherty, R. W. (1963). Physiological responses of swine to high concentrations of inhaled carbon dioxide. *Am. J. Vet. Res.* **24**, 329–332.

Norton, S., and Jewett, R. E. (1965a). Effect of drugs on spontaneous slow potential oscillations of the cerebral cortex. *J. Pharmacol. Exptl. Therap.* **149**, 301–310.

Norton, S., and Jewett, R. E. (1965b). Frequencies of slow potential oscillations in the cortex of cats. *Electroencephalog. Clin. Neurophysiol.* **19**, 377–386.

Opitz, E., and Schneider, M. (1950). Über die Sauerstoffversorgung des Gehirns und den Mechanismus von Mangelwirkungen. *Ergeb. Physiol. Biol. Chem. Exptl. Pharmakol.* **46**, 126–261.

Otomo, E. (1966). Beta wave activity in the electroencephalogram in cases of coma due to acute brain-stem lesions. *J. Neurol., Neurosurg., Psychiat.* [N. S.] **29**, 383–390.

Padel, Y., and Dell, P. (1965). Effets bulbaires et réticulaires des stimulations endormantes du tronc vago-aortique. *J. Physiol. (Paris)* **57**, 269–270.

Pagano, R. R., and Gault, F. P. (1964). Amygdala activity: A central measure of arousal. *Electroencephalog. Clin. Neurophysiol.* **17**, 255–260.

Pampiglione, G. (1963). "Development of Cerebral Function in the Dog." Butterworth, London and Washington, D.C.

Peñaloza-Rojas, J. H., Elterman, M., and Olmos, N. (1964). Sleep induced by cortical stimulation. *Exptl. Neurol.* **10**, 140–147.

Petersen, J., Di Perri, R., and Himwich, W. A. (1964). The comparative development of the EEG in rabbit, cat, and dog. *Electroencephalog. Clin. Neurophysiol.* **17**, 557–563.

Pick, E. P., and Miller, M. M. (1945). Influence of depletion of diffusable electrolytes upon electrical activity of the brain. *J. Neurophysiol.* **8**, 47–54.

Podvoll, E. M., and Goodman, S. J. (1967). Averaged neural electrical activity and arousal. *Science* **155**, 223–225.

Pollock, G. H. (1949). Central inhibitory effects of carbon dioxide. *J. Neurophysiol.* **12**, 315–324.

Pompeiano, O. (1963). EEG synchronization induced by peripheral nerve stimulation. *Prog. Brain Res.* 1, 429–443.

Pompeiano, O. (1967). The neurophysiological mechanisms of the postural and motor events during desynchronized sleep. Sleep and Altered States of Consciousness. *Proc. Assoc. Res. Nerve and Mental Disorders* 2, 351–423.

Prince, D. A., and Shanzer, S. (1966). Effects of anesthetics upon the EEG response to reticular stimulation. Patterns of slow synchrony. *Electroencephalog. Clin. Neurophysiol.* 21, 578–588.

Pscheidt, G. R., Steiner, W. G., and Himwich, H. E. (1963). An electroencephalographic and chemical re-evaluation of the central action of reserpine in the rabbit. *J. Pharmacol. Exptl. Therap.* 144, 37–44.

Roldan, E., and Escobar, A. (1961). Control de la actividad convulsiva y effecto sobre la transmission atrente producidos por el metaminodiazepoxido. Estudio experimental en el gato. *Bol. Inst. Estud. Med. Biol. (Mex.)* 19, 125–153.

Root, W. S., and Hofmann, F. G., eds. (1963). "Physiological Pharmacology." Vol. I. Academic Press, New York.

Rosomoff, H. L. (1960). Protective effects of hypothermia against pathological processes of the nervous system. *Ann. N.Y. Acad. Sci.* 80, 475–486.

Rossi, G. F., and Zanchetti, A. (1957). The brain stem reticular formation. Anatomy and physiology. *Arch. Ital. Biol.* 95, 199–438.

Rothballer, A. B. (1956). Studies on the adrenalin-sensitive component of the reticular activating system. *Electroencephalog. Clin. Neurophysiol.* 8, 603–621.

Rothballer, A. B. (1959). The effects of catecholamines on the central nervous system. *Pharmacol. Rev.* 11, 494–547.

Rowland, V., and Gluck, H. (1960). Electrographic arousal and its inhibition as studied by auditory conditioning. *Recent Advan. Biol. Psychiat., Proc. Ann. 14th Conv. Soc. Biol. Psychiat., Atlantic City, 1959* Vol. 2, pp. 96–105. Grune & Stratton, New York.

Rubin, M. A., Hoff, H. E., Winkler, A. W., and Smith, P. K. (1943). Intravenous potassium, calcium, magnesium and the cortical electrogram of the cat. *J. Neurophysiol.* 6, 23–28.

Runnals, S. (1962). Hyperventilation: An activating procedure in electroencephalography. *Am. J. EEG Technol.* 2, 9–18.

Sadowski, B., and Longo, V. G. (1962). Electroencephalographic and behavioral correlates of an instrumental reward conditioned response in rabbits. *Electroencephalog. Clin. Neurophysiol.* 14, 465–476.

Savoldi, F., Arrigo, A., Bolzani, L., and Cosi, V. (1965). Action électrophysiologique des substances antimonoaminoxy dasiques. *Schweiz. Arch. Neurol., Neurochir. Psychiat.* 95, 271–319.

Sawyer, C. H., Kawakami, M., Everett, J. W., and Markee, J. E. (1959). (Five manuscripts.) *Endocrinology* 65, 614.

Schade, J. P., and Pascoe, E. G. (1964). Maturational changes in cerebral cortex. III. *Prog. Brain Res.* 9, 132–154.

Schallek, W., and Walz, D. (1953). Effects of *d*-amphetamine on the electroencephalogram of the dog. *Proc. Soc. Exptl. Biol. Med.* 82, 715–719.

Schlag, J. D., and Chaillet, F. (1962). Thalamic mechanisms involved in cortical desynchronization and recruiting responses. *Electroencephalog. Clin. Neurophysiol.* 15, 39–62.

Schweigerdt, A. K., Stewart, A. H., and Himwich, H. E. (1966). An electrographic study of *d*-lysergic acid diethylamide and nine congeners. *J. Pharmacol. Exptl. Therap.* 151, 353–359.

Shimizu, A., Hishikawa, Y., Matsumoto, K., and Kaneko, Z. (1964). Electroencephalographic studies on the action of monoamine oxidase inhibitor. *Psychopharmacology* **6**, 368–387.

Smith, P. K., Winkler, A. W., and Hoff, H. E. (1942). The pharmacological action of parenterally administered magnesium salts; A review. *Anesthesiology* **3**, 323–330.

Spoerel, W. E. (1962). The electroencephalogram after cardiac arrest. *Can. Anaesth. Soc. J.* **9**, 479–487.

Spooner, C. E., and Winters, W. D. (1966). Intra-arterial blood pressure recording in the unrestrained check during wakefulness and sleep. *Arch. Intern. Pharmacodyn.* **161**, 1–6.

Spooner, C. E., and Winters, W. D. (1967). The influence of centrally active amine induced blood pressure changes on the electroencephalogram and behavior. *Intern. J. Neuropharmacol.* **6**, 109–118.

Starzl, T. E., Taylor, C. W., and Magoun, H. W. (1951). Ascending conduction in reticular activating system with special reference to the diencephalon. *J. Neurophysiol.* **14**, 461–477.

Steiner, J. E., and Sulman, F. G. (1963). Simultaneous studies of blood sugar, behavioral changes and EEG on the awake rabbit after administration of psilocybin. *Arch. Intern. Pharmacodyn.* **145**, 301–308.

Sterman, M. B., and Clemente, C. D. (1962). Forebrain inhibitory mechanisms: Cortical synchronization induced by forebrain stimulation. *Exptl. Neurol.* **6**, 91–102; refer also to pp. 103–117.

Stern, J. A., Ulett, G. A., and Sines, J. O. (1960). Electrocortical changes during conditioning. *Recent Advan. Biol. Psychiat., Proc. Ann. 14th Conv. Soc. Biol. Psychiat., Atlantic City, 1959* Vol. 2, pp. 106–122. Grune & Stratton, New York.

Stumpf, C. (1965). The fast component in the electrical activity of rabbit's hippocampus. *Electroencephalog. Clin. Neurophysiol.* **18**, 477–486.

Sugar, O., and Gerard, R. (1938). Anoxia and brain potentials. *J. Neurophysiol.* **1**, 558–572.

Swank, R. L., and Watson, C. W. (1949). Effects of barbiturates and anesthesia on spontaneous electrical activity of dog brain. *J. Neurophysiol.* **12**, 137–160.

Toman, J. E. P. (1952). Neuropharmacology of peripheral nerve. *Pharmacol. Rev.* **4**, 168–218.

Toman, J. E. P., and Davis, J. P. (1949). The effects of drugs upon the electrical activity of the brain. *Pharmacol. Rev.* **1**, 425–492.

Twente, J. W., and Twente, J. A. (1965). Effects of core temperature upon duration of hibernation of *Citellus lateralis. J. Appl. Physiol.* **20**, 411–416.

Valtax, J. L., Jouvet, D., and Jouvet, M. (1964). Evolution électroencephographique des différents états de sommeil chez le chaton. *Electroencephalog. Clin. Neurophysiol.* **17**, 218–233.

Weinberger, N., Yeudall, L., and Lindsley, D. B. (1968). EEG correlates of reinforced behavioral inhibition. *Psychon. Sci.* **10**, 11–12.

Wells, C. E. (1963). Electroencephalographic correlates of conditioned responses. *In* "EEG and Behavior" (G. H. Glaser, ed.), pp. 60–108. Basic Books, New York.

White, R. P., and Daigneault, E. A. (1959). The antagonism of atropine to the EEG effects of adrenergic drugs. *J. Pharmacol. Exptl. Therap.* **125**, 339–346.

Winters, W. D., Mori, K., Spooner, C. E., and Bauer, R. O. (1967). The neurophysiology of anesthesia. *Anesthesiology* **28**, 65–80.

Woodbury, D. M. (1952). Effect of adrenocortical steroids and adrenocorticotrophic hormone on electroshock seizure threshold. *J. Pharmacol. Exptl. Therap.* **105**, 27–36.

Woodbury, D. M. (1958). Relation between the adrenal cortex and the central nervous system. *Pharmacol. Rev.* **10**, 275–357.

Woodbury, D. M., Rollins, L. T., Garnder, M. D., Hirschi, W. L., Hogan, J. R., Rallison, M. L., Tanner, G. S., and Brodie, D. A. (1958). Effects of carbon dioxide on brain excitability and electrolytes. *Am. J. Physiol.* **192**, 79–90.

Woolley, D. E., and Timiras, P. S. (1962). The gonad-brain relationship effects of female sex hormones on electroshock convulsions in the rat. *Endocrinology* **70**, 196–209.

Wurtz, R. H. (1965). Steady potential shifts during arousal and deep sleep in the cat. *Electroencephalog. Clin. Neurophysiol.* **18**, 649–662.

Yamaguchi, N., Ling, G. M., and Marczynski, T. J. (1964). Recruiting responses observed during wakefulness and sleep in unanesthetized chronic cats. *Electroencephalog. Clin. Neurophysiol.* **17**, 246–254.

7

EEG Correlates of Pathologic Changes

∽ I. "Epilepsy"

A brief discussion of the human disease epilepsy seems appropriate, because it should clarify the later discussions on experimentally produced and naturally occurring epilepsy in animals. Basically, epilepsy refers to conditions in which the patient has convulsions accompanied by various EEG changes of unusual waveforms, usually of large amplitude.

Epilepsy is often produced by inflammatory or destructive lesions in the brain that result from various infectious and noninfectious causes. Some human epilepsy occurs in which no organic lesions can be found, so-called "idiopathic" or "cryptogenic" epilepsy; biochemical lesions are the most probable cause.

Clinical epilepsy in humans has been conventionally classified into 2 main types: (1) In *petit mal* there are convulsions and brief lapses of consciousness; the EEG contains characteristic paroxysmal patterns of paired spikes and waves of about 3/sec (Fig. 7-1). There is also a petit mal variant EEG type that occurs in children 2–5 years old (Fig. 7-2). (2) In *grand mal* there are generalized tonic–clonic convulsions, often violent, and the EEG contains erratic, relatively fast, high-voltage activity (Fig. 7-3).

This simple scheme, however, is incomplete because various people consider many other types of bizarre EEGs to indicate epilepsy. This is

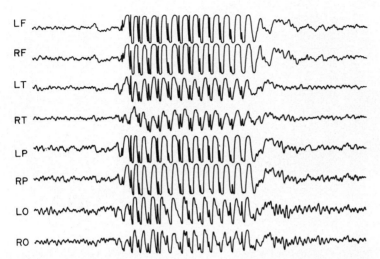

Fig. 7-1. Petit mal EEG in the human. LF and RF, left and right frontal; LT and RT, left and right temporal; LP and RP, left and right parietal; and LO and RO, left and right occipital. (Sadove *et al.*, 1967.)

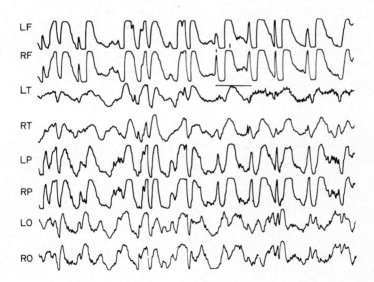

Fig. 7-2. Petit mal variant EEG in the human. Abbreviations are the same as in Fig. 7-1. (Sadove *et al.*, 1967.)

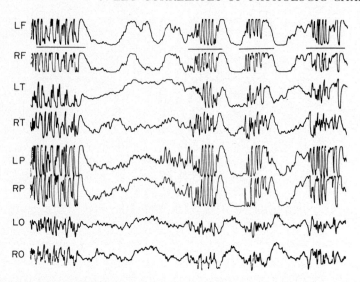

FIG. 7-3.   Grand mal EEG in the human. Abbreviations are the same as in Fig. 7-1.
(Sadove *et al.*, 1967.)

illustrated by the variety of techniques that have been used in animals
to experimentally simulate epilepsy. For example, although penicillin,
alumina cream, and strychnine are commonly used, more than 58
chemicals have been used either systematically or topically to produce
experimental epilepsy (reviewed by Ajmone Marsan, 1965, 1966). In
addition, many studies in animals have employed strong, repetitive
electric stimulation of the brain to induce motor and electrographic
seizures.

These conditions produce various types of "epileptiform" EEG activity, and it is doubtful that they all act by similar mechanisms. It therefore
is unlikely that all provide experimental models of epilepsy that are
equally valid (Ajmone Marsan, 1965).

For the sake of simplicity, we could define epilepsy as follows: *any
convulsive motor disorder associated with bizarre electric activity*. This definition, however, raises questions about the limits of "bizarre." Inspection
of published EEG records that authors designate as epileptiform, or
simply seizures, reveals a great variety of waveforms. Activity that most
people would call bizarre can occur without a convulsive accompaniment, as during anesthesia of diseased animals (refer to Fig. 7-8) or
during animal hypnosis when animals are treated with certain seizure-
inducing drugs (refer to Fig. 6-11b). These complications emphasize the
ambiguities that arise in any attempt to define epilepsy. From a clinical
point of view, there seems to be no special advantage to using the term
epilepsy for animals, because convulsions can result from a wide variety

of diseases. In fact, the term probably should not be used at all, because to some people it misleadingly connotes a condition of genetic origin.

With these admittedly hazy notions in mind, we can now consider studies in which lesions have been produced. These studies[1] are important because they indicate something about the genesis, time course, and electrographic correlates of brain lesions.

II. Experimentally Produced Brain Disease

Most studies have been made by creating a discrete lesion that then becomes a focus for the generation of EEG seizures. Although the seizures often are limited by a surrounding zone of inhibitory neurons, spread is possible. Sometimes the spread is to contralateral homotopic regions, creating what is called a "mirror focus." Discharges also can spread to involve the entire brain.

Seizures do not always arise spontaneously as a consequence of a focal lesion, either artificially produced or naturally occurring. Various techniques are used, experimentally or clinically, to "activate" a seizure. These include repetitive sensory stimulation of certain sensory paths (auditory or visual). Seizures can also be activated by stimulant drugs, carbon dioxide, sleep, and anesthetics.

A. Chemically Induced Abnormalities

Petit mal epilepsy is very difficult to simulate, but there are several reports that describe its artificial induction. One of these involved the use of a quinazolone derivative that produced electrographic and behavioral signs like those occurring in petit mal epilepsy (Morillo and Baylor, 1964). Another method involves low-frequency stimulation of nonspecific thalamic nuclei in cats as they awaken from light anesthesia; under such conditions normal recruiting responses can change into a spike and wave response (Pollen *et al.*, 1964; also see below).

Most artificially produced lesions cause variations of grand mal epilepsy. Topical application of penicillin to neural tissue is one of the common methods of simulating epilepsy. The usual consequence is paroxysms of electrographic spikes and sharp waves that begin a few minutes after application. During the ictal[2] periods the paroxysms are

---

[1]The most comprehensive review of such studies is the well-illustrated work of Kriendler (1965; refer also to Ajmone Marsan, 1965, 1966).

[2]Ictal periods are usually defined to mean periods when rhythmic, self-sustaining electrographic discharges and motor seizures occur, whereas during interictal periods convulsive activity is either absent or isolated. Electrographic abnormalities, however, often occur during interictal periods.

quite prominent, whereas only isolated spikes occur interictally. Even though a lesion may be focal, during ictal periods the abnormal electric or activity may spread to involve most of the brain. One study with penicillin (Rovit and Swiecicki, 1965) revealed that epileptiform discharges in a focus could spread to the contralateral homotopic areas. They also observed that 2 independent penicillin foci could facilitate each other, especially when the foci were symmetrically located in opposite hemispheres. The mutual facilitating effect of 2 foci was indicated by a faster rate of spike discharge and by a wider distribution of EEG abnormality. Such results agree with human clinical observations in which surgical removal of one abnormal focus sometimes results in diminished seizure tendencies in another, presumably independent, focus. The major conclusion seems to be that if 2 foci are synaptically connected in a relatively direct way, seizure discharges can be transmitted from either area to the other. Eventually each formerly discrete focus fires more and more frequently and more independently.

Alumina cream is also used to induce experimental epilepsy. In such a study in rabbits by Visser (1962), cortical injections of alumina produced focal HVSA, spikes, and sharp waves. Auditory stimulation, instead of augmenting the abnormality, actually abolished it. The general level of excitement seemed to suppress abnormality, and for some time after animals were brought from the animal room to the laboratory the EEG appeared normal. These findings suggest that relaxed states can *disinhibit* abnormal foci. Verification comes from the observations that maximal alumina-induced abnormality occurred during sleep (Chow and Obrist, 1954). Likewise, sleep augments epileptic discharges in humans (Sadove *et al.*, 1967) and anesthesia enhances such discharges in some animals (Klemm and Mallo, 1966).

The study in which Dow *et al.* (1962) used cortical implants of cobalt powder to induce epilepsy in rats revealed an initial "delta" activity,[3] followed in a few days by additional development of isolated sharp waves. Thereafter the sharp waves tended to occur in bursts. A few days later the EEG rhythm had returned to a more normal state, but bursts of large voltage spikes were evident. Initially the EEG abnormalities appeared only in bipolar arrangements in which one electrode was near the focus. Later abnormalities spread intracortically in many rats. During the recovery period of 4–6 weeks after cobalt application, the spike amplitudes and frequencies decreased. Although the lesions were always made in the right frontal cortex, both repetitive photostimulation

---

[3]This term, commonly used in human electroencephalography, is introduced to indicate an abnormal degree of HVSA. It usually refers to frequencies slower than about 3–4/sec.

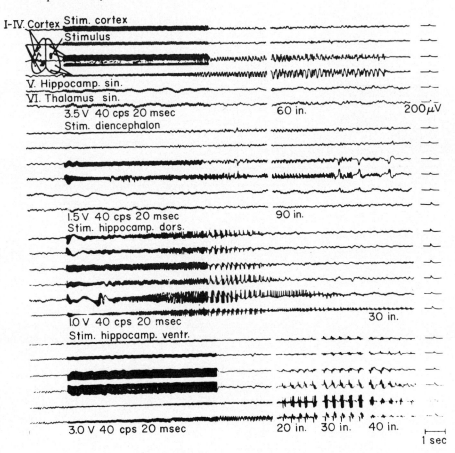

FIG. 7-4. Electrographic afterdischarge following 40/sec electric stimulation of cortex, lateral thalamus (Diencephalon), and dorsal (Hippocamp. Dors.) and ventral hippocampus (Hippocamp. Ventr.). First 4 traces (I–IV) were recorded from the cortex, while the bottom 2 (V–VI) were recorded from the hippocampus and thalamus. (Monnier and Gangloff, 1961.)

and audiostimulation greatly enhanced epileptiform activity when the stimulation was prolonged.

In a study of anesthetic effects on experimentally produced epilepsy, Coceani *et al.* (1966) found that cortical epileptiform discharges produced by penicillin were depressed by perfusion of the areas with amobarbital (average dose of 10 mg). This depression was prevented by breathing 5% CO_2 in air. Foci outside but near the border of perfused areas were not depressed and sometimes were even activated by amobarbital. Amobarbital did not suppress diffuse epileptiform activity induced by intraventricular penicillin or by intravenous chlorambucil.

B. ELECTRICALLY INDUCED ABNORMALITIES

Direct cortical stimulation is another way to induce epileptiform activity (Straw and Mitchell, 1966). Stimulus threshold varies with species, site of stimulation, and stimulus parameters. The characteristic response to sufficiently intense stimuli is an afterdischarge that persists for a few milliseconds to several minutes.

Electrically induced cortical afterdischarges often occur in a definite sequence of successive stages: brief desynchrony, rhythmic synchronous discharges, interrupted clonic discharge, isoelectric "exhaustion," and HVSA during recovery (reviewed by Kriendler, 1965). Intense stimulation of subcortical areas also will induce epileptiform afterdischarge in those areas. Some of these changes are illustrated in Fig. 7-4.

C. SURGICALLY INDUCED ABNORMALITIES

Aside from stimulating properties of electric current, intense stimulation destroys neural tissue, and the sequelae of strategically placed lesions could lead to improved understanding of neuropathologic processes.

Although relatively few such studies have been conducted, in recent years such studies have improved our understanding of cortical spindling changes that occur in disease. Although spindles often accompany delta activity, they may be generated independently. Evidence for such a conclusion includes the presence of spindles without delta waves in *cerveau isolé* cats or during barbiturate anesthesia. On the other hand, large doses of ethyl alcohol produce prominent delta waves with only rare spindles (Kogi *et al.*, 1960).

In a study of subcortical mechanisms that generate cortical delta activity, Nakamura and Ohye (1964) produced discrete lesions in various regions of midpontine, pretrigeminal sectioned cats. They found that bilateral destruction of the posterior hypothalamus induced generalized cortical spindles and delta activity, along with hippocampal spiking. Arousing stimuli delivered to the nonspecific thalamic projection areas abolished spindles without affecting delta activity, whereas stimulation of specific thalamic projection nuclei abolished delta activity without affecting spindles. Unilateral destruction of the posterior hypothalamus produced delta activity in the ipsilateral hemisphere. Following post-collicular section in the midpontine preparations, spindles appeared without delta activity. Unilateral destruction of specific thalamic projection areas induced an ipsilateral delta activity localized to the projection area without spindles; however, spindles became prominent, along with delta activity, if cats were also deprived of vision. Taken together these results suggest that afferent impulses in the posterior hypothalamus normally suppress both delta activity and spindles. Delta activity seems to be suppressed via activated specific thalamic nuclei, whereas spindles are suppressed via activated nonspecific thalamic relays.

D. Effects on Individual Neuron Functions

Several studies have correlated neuronal action potential properties with EEG epileptiform activity. These studies provide important information about the neural mechanisms. Epilepsy, usually being associated with excessive motor activity and large amplitude spikes or sharp waves, suggests hyperactivity of certain neurons. Recordings of action potentials have shown this to be true; but as we shall see later, sometimes neurons are underactive during epilepsy.

Penicillin-induced paroxysms in anesthetized cats produced active seizure periods in which extracellularly recorded action potentials had long durations and positive polarity and were associated with slow positive waves. During interictal periods, isolated EEG abnormalities were associated with bursts of action potentials that were diphasic and often progressively decreased in amplitude. These various changes were not observed with intracellular microelectrodes, and their explanation, yet to be established, may involve changes in size of the discharging epileptic cells and consequent changes in distance from the recording electrode (Matsumoto and Ajmone Marsan, 1964).

Another extracellular microelectrode study of convulsive activity was performed by Feher *et al.* (1965), who used topical applications of strychnine or *d*-tubocurarine to induce cortical epileptiform activity. Repetitive auditory stimulation evoked large triphasic EEG waves consisting of an initial small, positive wave, a second large, negative wave, and a final slow, positive wave. Simultaneous recording of the same potentials at deeper levels of the cortex revealed a polarity reversal, indicative of "dendritic" origin (Chapter I, Section II, A). Simultaneous unit recording revealed bursts of 1–5 action potentials in cortical neurons at the time of the initial fast positive component of the evoked epileptiform activity.

Evoked responses became afterdischarges of EEG spikes and sharp waves if the cortex also were treated with eserine and acetylcholine. EEG abnormalities apparently were generated in deep cortical layers, because there were no distinct polarity reversals between the surface and

deep regions. These afterdischarges were quite similar to the paroxsy-
mal activity in human epilepsy, in morphology, and in the character of
associated muscle activity. The discharges were associated with bursts of
unit activity. During the onset of the first EEG spike a relatively long
train of unit discharges occurred, while during the consecutive spikes
only shorter trains of 1–2 discharges occurred. The time relations between surface EEG potentials and unit potentials were strictly determined. If a unit began to fire during the positive phase of an EEG spike,
the consecutive discharges appeared in exact phase with the surface
negative waves.

These findings suggest an explanation for the mechanism of rhythmic
cortical afterpotentials. Discharges that originate in deep cortical
layers may conduct through vertically conducting neurons to the surface, whereupon surface neurons discharge and reexcite the deeper
neurons, establishing reverberatory circuits for self-sustained activity.

Particularly interesting are studies that have analyzed neuronal activity during the spike and wave discharges of simulated petit mal. These
EEG patterns are actually a modified form of recruiting that can be
produced in cats by 3/sec stimulation of nonspecific thalamic nuclei
during a critical period of recovery from carefully controlled light
anesthesia. AC-amplifier recording from extracellular microelectrodes
revealed that unit activity increased during the surface spike but was depressed during the surfacd slow wave (Fig. 7-5). The cessation of unit
activity is attributed to long-lasting IPSPs occurring in deep regions
(Pollen *et al.*, 1964). IPSPs have been associated with extracellular
positivity, and when these occur deeply they cause the surface to become
relatively negative. Thus, petit mal probably has inhibitory components
that are inoperative during the grand mal type of epilepsy. IPSPs
also might be suppressed by excessive anesthesia, and this could explain why the slow EEG component appears only during a critical stage
of anesthesia.

Intracellular recordings during EEG seizures have revealed that action potential bursts associated with EEG spikes result from sudden,
excessive depolarizations of the membrane. The 2 most striking features
of such paroxsmal depolarizations are their excessive degree and
relatively long duration.

Such studies also revealed an interesting enhancement of MP oscillations (refer to Chapter 1, Section I, C; Fig. 7-6). These oscillations are
associated with action potential discharge on the depolarizing phase, but
the magnitude of the slow change is much greater than that which occurs
normally. Such phenomena were studied in anesthetized cats subjected
to topical cortical applications of penicillin; the intracellular changes

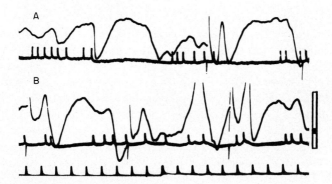

FIG. 7-5. Spike and wave EEG responses (upper trace of each pair) induced by 3/sec electric stimulation of the intralaminar thalamus of a cat in a critical stage of arousal from anesthesia. Simultaneous extracellular microelectrode recording from the same area of cortex (lower trace of each pair) revealed that unit discharges stopped during the long duration EEG waves. Same unit in A and B, but separated by 5 min. In B, when stimulation failed to evoke the large surface slow wave, unit fired randomly. Positivity is upward in each channel. Calibrations: 150 μV (surface), 10 mV (unit); 50 msec time marks shown at bottom. (Pollen *et al.*, 1964.)

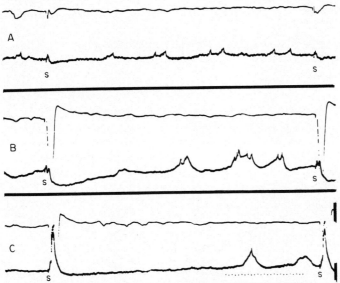

FIG. 7-6. Activation of penicillin-induced epileptic focus by electric stimulations of contralateral homologous cortex. Upper trace of each pair is surface activity recorded from gross electrodes; lower trace is intracellular activity from a cell in the same region. A: Before topical application of penicillin; B: about 3 min after penicillin; C: about 5 min after B. Upward deflections in both traces indicate positivity. Stimulus strength in A and B = 1.5 times that of C. Calibrations: 1 mV (upper trace), 10 mV (lower trace), and 50 cps. (Matsumoto, 1964.)

occurred spontaneously and could also be evoked by appropriate electrical stimulation of the focus (Matsumoto, 1964). When the MP oscillations were very large, they were always associated with spike activity in the EEG.

In similar studies, Sawa *et al.* (1965) observed that penicillin applications ultimately decreased IPSPs and simultaneously caused summation of EPSPs. They also discussed and illustrated the sustained MP depolarization which occurs during seizure episodes. Electric stimulation during seizures elicited EPSPs but not IPSPs, indicating depression of IPSP mechanisms during this type of seizure. Enhanced EPSPs and depressed IPSPs presumably act synergistically to produce epileptic seizures. Furthermore, at the end of a seizure episode, EPSPs could no longer be induced by electric stimulation, suggesting that seizures terminate spontaneously when EPSP phenomena become inoperative.

The relations between IPSPs and EPSPs are considered by Ajmone Marsan (1965) to determine whether the epilepsy is ictal or interictal. Intracellular recordings reveal a mixture of IPSPs and EPSPs associated with interictal phenomena. However, when IPSPs disappear, EPSPs superimposed on a sustained depolarization dominate and organized ictal periods are likely to start. Thus, maximal seizure activity has been shown at the cell level to result from disinhibition.

All the research on artificially produced electrographic seizures has proved several points:

1. Epilepsy results from excessive neuronal discharges that are often augmented by disinhibition.
2. A focal seizure, if intense enough, can recruit healthy neurons into abnormal discharge and result in generalized seizures.
3. Seizures can be generated from a cortical or subcortical focus.
4. Two or more focal seizures can be generated independently, with or without interaction.
5. A given cortical focus occasionally may be represented by a mirror focus in the contralateral homotopic cortex.

Useful as this information is, it is limited to epilepsy. Unfortunately, many if not most neural disorders in animals are not epilepsy. Many of these conditions, such as tumors, encephalitis, and vascular disorders, are discussed in detail later. Additionally, 2 major categories of nonepileptic brain disease occur as part of irradiation and nutritional deficiency syndromes. Anoxia could be considered yet another category, but it is discussed elsewhere (Chapter 6, Section III, A).

III. Naturally Occurring Brain Disease

Relatively few EEG studies have been conducted in animals with naturally occurring brain disease.[4] Unlike human electroencephalography, there is no accumulation of observations over several decades. All that will be attempted here is to summarize the present state of the art and hope that more useful knowledge will be obtained in the near future. One of the main reasons for writing the book was to provide technical background and stimulation for more investigators to pursue comparative and veterinary medical electroencephalography.

A. EEG SIGNS OF LESIONS

Pathologic processes invariably manifest themselves in abnormal neuronal electric activity. These abnormalities may be classified in the following oversimplified way:

> Spikes and sharp waves
> High voltage, fast activity (HVFA)
> High voltage, slow activity (HVSA)
> Low voltage, fast activity (LVFA)
> Spindle abnormalities

These abnormalities may appear alone or in combination. Spikes or HVFA may exaggerate to become epileptiform seizures. All types may appear persistently or paroxysmally.

The first problem in EEG analysis is to determine whether or not EEG patterns are abnormal. Although this is often obvious, subtle abnormalities may go undetected unless a clear idea exists as to what is normal. There are only a few reports of EEG studies in normal dogs, with electrode arrangements that would be used clinically; the normal EEG in unanesthetized dogs is described by Redding (1965) and that in anesthetized dogs by Klemm (1968a). Much more information is needed on clinically normal animals.

B. LOCALIZATION OF LESIONS

After EEG abnormality is detected in one or more leads, it is important to identify the neural origin of these abnormal potentials. The initial question to answer is this: Is the brain pathology focal or diffuse?

---

[4]For basic information on animal neurology, the reader is referred to the books by McGrath (1960), Palmer (1965), and Hoerlein (1965).

The answer is not always obvious from EEG examination.[5] If abnormal potentials appear in several leads, they could have arisen from one focus. Amplitudes may be decreased at electrodes that are most distant from the focus. Usually identification of an isolated focus requires bipolar techniques, in which one takes advantage of amplifier polarity connections to assist in localization. The process is called triangulation; although it need not involve a triangular field, it does require simultaneous recording on 2 channels from 3 electrodes, one of which is common to the input of both channels (Fig. 7-7). If we assume in the figure that the anterior electrode is numbered 3, the left occipital 4, and the right occipital 5, then the electrode pairs are 3-4, 4-5, and 5-3. An abnormal discharge that arises under site 4 would appear in both leads connected to 4 (and perhaps in other leads too); however, the direction of the discharge, + or −, will be out of phase in the 2 recordings. The reason is that in the top record, electrode 4 is connected to the positive amplifier input and, in the middle record, electrode 4 is connected to the negative input. Similar reasoning applies to the conclusion that the records also indicate a lesion at electrode 5.

C. EEG as a Basis for Diagnosis and Prognosis

Study of the EEG one day may be as clinically useful in animal medicine as it is in human medicine. It is obvious from the previous discussion that more information is needed.

A major problem is the lack of standardization of technique in veterinary electroencephalography. Some of the basic issues involved were discussed in a publication by Klemm (1968c).

The major issue is the method of restraint. Some means of restraint is absolutely essential, even in cooperative animals. Muscle and motion potential artifacts, when present, often preclude sensible analysis. Many animals can be made to lie still, although temporal muscle potential artifacts persist unless local anesthesia is used. Even during general anesthesia, temporal muscle spasms occur, although they do tend to be transient except in the lightest stages of anesthesia (refer to Figs. 3-10 and 7-9).

Redding's technique (1964) of restraint requires binding of the feet, covering eyes, plugging ears, anesthetizing temporal muscles, and holding animals in lateral recumbency until struggling stops. Another technique involves the use of paralyzing doses of the muscle relaxant gallamine (Herin et al., 1968). My own technique involves the use of sodium pentobarbital or sodium pentothal, in light anesthesic doses (Stage III, Plane 1 or 2, Guedel scheme).

[5]Further explanation on identifying the origin of a focus is presented in Chapter V.

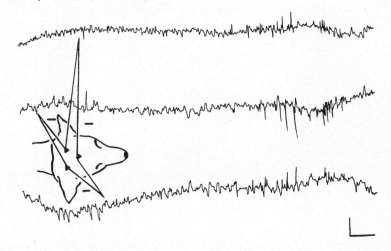

Fig. 7-7. Illustration of triangulation technique for localizing lesions in the brain. Negative signs indicate which lead of each pair is connected to the negative amplifier input. Out-of-phase spikes in the top 2 recordings indicate a lesion arising from the electrode common to both leads. Likewise, out-of-phase spikes in the bottom 2 traces indicate a lesion at the common electrode. The lesion in this dog is over both occipital regions. Calibrations: 50 μV; 1 sec. (Klemm and Mallo, 1966.)

Each of these 3 restraint methods has serious limitations, which are summarized in Table 7-1. The LVFA present in the EEG of conscious dogs is difficult to analyze because the magnitude is only 0–20 μV (Herin *et al.*, 1968; Redding and Colwell, 1964). The discrepancies in the various reports (Herin *et al.*, 1968) on frequency content of normal EEGs may be due in large measure to the difficulty of analyzing low-amplitude waveforms.

Mixed arousal and sleep patterns create some interpretation difficulties because 2 frames of reference are needed for comparison with normal EEGs. Both states are valuable because they are more "physiologic" than drugged states. Sleep also can activate EEG abnormalities (Redding, 1965). In the study of hydrocephalus by deLahunta and Cummings (1965), 2 of the 3 dogs had near normal EEGs when they were awake.

Sleep also activates some EEG abnormalities in man (F. A. Gibbs *et al.*, 1947; Gibbs and Gibbs, 1965). Anesthesia (sodium thiopental) is used to record from children and in recording in adults when sphenoidal electrodes are used. Although a degree of HVSA results, signs of lesions are still evident (Hill and Parr, 1963). Another ultrashort acting barbiturate, methohexital, has also been recommended for EEG studies of children (Frank *et al.*, 1966).

TABLE 7-1
DISADVANTAGES OF 3 MEANS OF RESTRAINING ANIMALS FOR EEG RECORDING[a]

Disadvantages	Manual (no drugs)	Muscle relaxants	Anesthesia
Muscle artifact	X	–	–
Motion artifact	X	–	–
Time-consuming	X	X	–
Low voltages, difficult analysis	X	X	–
Mixed arousal, sleep; interpretation problems	X	X	–
Poor contrast between awake electro-encephalogram and abnormal low voltage–fast activity	X	X	–
No activation by disinhibition	X	X	–
Hospitalization required	–	–	X
Hazardous	–	X	X
Masking of encephalographic abnormalities?	X	X	X

[a]Klemm (1968c).

Abnormal LVFA occurs commonly and may be best demonstrated in anesthetized animals (Klemm, 1968b). Thus, this is one example of how an *alert* state can mask abnormality. Another example is that active inhibitory processes during alert states can suppress abnormality. Activation of EEG abnormality by disinhibition can occur during sleep and anesthesia.

Although anesthetics have long been considered neural depressants, recent multiple-unit studies in cats reveal that this depression is only partial; in fact, some units may become more active by disinhibition (Goodman and Mann, 1967). These observations applied even to portions of the midbrain reticular formation, previously thought to be selectively depressed by anesthetics.

Anesthesia, due to its disinhibiting abilities, can occasionally trigger electrographic seizures. Bizarre activity (spikes, HVFA, and HVSA) was noted in 10 dogs and 1 cat. An illustration of the seizures of 4 of these animals is shown in Fig. 7-8. Since that time many other anesthetized dogs have exhibited electrographic seizures, some of which were much more extreme than those illustrated.

Anesthetized dogs and, to a lesser extent, paralyzed dogs, require hospitalization because of the prolonged recovery time from the drug. Ultrashort anesthetics are not convenient because they do not provide a long recording period or a stable EEG; these drugs, however, are safer to use in high-risk cases. Hospitalization has not proved to be much of a practical problem, because patients are often referred to the university clinic for other observations and testing.

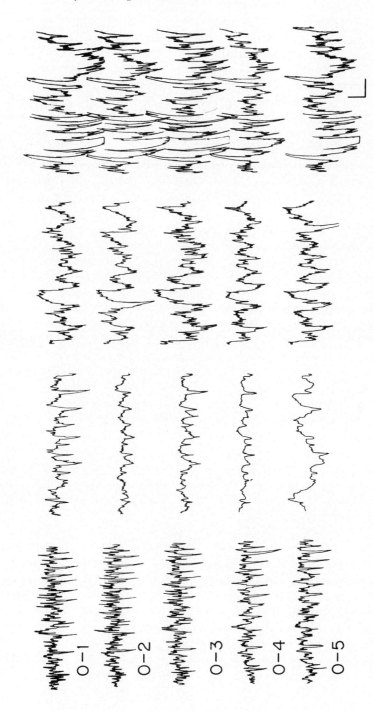

Fig. 7-8. Examples of brain seizure activity recorded from 4 different anesthetized dogs. 0 = reference site on nose; 1 = left frontal; 2 = right frontal; 3 = vertex; 4 = left occipital; and 5 = right occipital. Calibrationns: 100 μV; 1 sec.

Both muscle relaxants and anesthesia are potentially dangerous. Failure to achieve rapid tracheal intubation and resuscitation can cause death from muscle paralysis. Also, forced breathing can fatally retard venous return in cardiovascular patients. Anesthesia can cause respiratory or cardiac failure; and patients should be intubated and observed closely by an attendant during EEG recording. There is no indication yet that anesthesia is contraindicated for purely central nervous system diseases. Many extremely ill patients, some with added cardiovascular complications, have tolerated anesthesia well.

Muscle relaxants, by deafferentiation, create an unphysiologic condition, and thus could mask EEG abnormality. There is a possibility of EEG interpretation ambiguities resulting from such variables as catecholamine release in frightened dogs and CO_2 blood level changes during forced respiration. These possibilities have not been proved, however. Paralyzed dogs generally display HVSA, but this can be converted into arousal-type EEGs by visual and auditory stimulation (Herin *et al.*, 1968).

Possible masking of EEG abnormality by anesthetic is a major reason why others hesitate to use this method of restraint. There is no doubt that light anesthesia produces the general effect, *in normal animals*, of high amplitude, slow EEG frequencies, and spindles. The *relevant* question, however, is whether anesthesia masks EEG abnormalities in diseased animals and, if so, does that masking prevent diagnosis. Such masking is commonly assumed, but not really supported by any published evidence. Anesthetized normal dogs had stable EEG patterns (Klemm, 1968a) that were distinctly different in any 10-min recording period from that of more than 160 anesthetized patients studied. All of the usual signs of abnormality (spikes, sharp waves, LVFA, and HVSA) have been observed during anesthesia. Moreover, abnormal LVFA, sharp waves, and spindle abnormalities are more apparent during anesthesia, indicating that in this sense anesthesia causes less masking than does alert wakefulness.

Direct comparisons, with and without anesthesia, have been reported (Klemm and Mallo, 1966). The abnormalities that were evident without anesthesia were also evident with anesthesia. Due to reduced artifacts, EEGs obtained under anesthesia were more readily interpreted (Fig. 7-9). In the records of the dog that is not illustrated, signs of lesions could not be distinguished from artifact without anesthesia. During anesthesia, an initial generalized brain seizure activity occurred, followed by an interictal period which contained HVSA.

My own conclusions about the present-day utility of EEG studies are based on data from anesthetized animals. This has resulted in confusion,

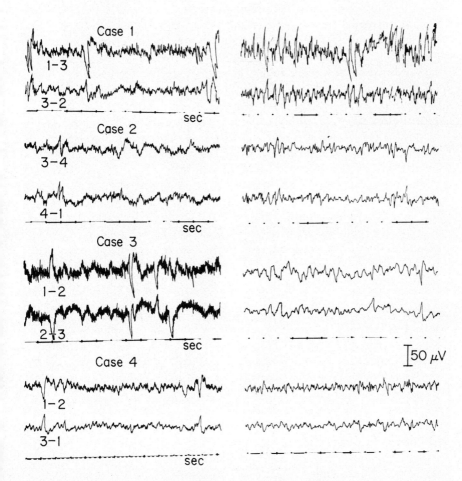

FIG. 7-9. EEGs of 4 dogs illustrating localized signs of HVSA when unanesthetized (left) and when the same dog was subsequently anesthetized (right). The bipolar records were taken from sites that had abnormal waveforms in previous monopolar recordings. Localization of lesion is indicated by HVSA that is out of phase. Many of the apparently abnormal waves on the left are probably affected by respiratory movements (heavy portion of 1-sec time mark lines), whereas under anesthesia these abnormal waves cannot be suspected as artifact. The high-frequency spikes in the records of case 3, unanesthetized, are muscle potentials. The spikes in the record of case 1 can be attributed to neural origin on the basis of their prominence during anesthesia. Numbers refer to the same electrode sites as in Fig. 7-8. (Klemm and Mallo, 1966.)

as other workers have preferred to use unanesthetized animals. Although there are many examples given that illustrate the same basic EEG abnormality in a given disease, with or without anesthesia, it is unwise to generalize freely. Anesthesia may cause brain lesions to manifest themselves in a different pattern of EEG abnormality. This is certainly true in those cases in which seizures are "triggered" by the abnormality.

Evidence to date gives little grounds for hoping to associate a given EEG abnormality with a given disease. Rather, it seems that the most dependable information obtainable from the EEG is *presence of abnormality, type of abnormality, distribution of abnormality,* and *severity of abnormality.* This information seems to be available from an EEG, whether or not it was derived under anesthesia.

The initial interpretation of EEG records is best done without any prior knowledge of case history of symptoms. This approach minimizes bias, so that the interpreter does not try to "see" things in the record that are not really there or to overlook important features in the EEG.[6] The EEG should be reinterpreted in the light of clinical findings. EEG examination may suggest several causes of the disease that may be distinguished on the basis of clinical information.

An abnormality usually takes the form of a change in frequency or amplitude. This conclusion is justified from both human and animal data. Such abnormalities indicate brain disease, although sometimes neither gross nor microscopic lesions are evident. Failure to demonstrate microscopic lesions may indicate that (1) the search was not extensive enough (sample size of histologic sections was too small) or (2) the lesion was biochemical and did not have visual manifestations.

Presence of *subtle* EEG abnormalities is easily detected when the abnormalities occur focally. Thus, distinct dissimilarities appear between symmetrically placed electrodes.

It is clear that a given type of abnormality, or any combination thereof, is seldom a reliable indicator of a specific disease. A certain type of EEG abnormality could indicate the general category of disease: (1) infection, (2) vascular disorder (hemorrhage or infarct), (3) tumor, or (4) trauma. As will be seen, these hopes are incompletely realized. *The various signs of lesions have more value in suggesting whether the disease is predominantly inflammatory or degenerative.* This point is confounded by complex relations between diseased tissue and the electric activity it generates. Some forms of pathology, such as necrosis or neoplasia of nonneural tissue, are electrically inert. Such disease is often indicated by a focal flattening of the EEG. Due to the wide spacing be-

---

[6] The electroencephalographer also should be tested occasionally by having him examine a *normal* dog that he has been told is a patient.

tween electrodes it is possible to miss detection of electrically silent areas. The EEG from regions immediately adjacent to the lesion may reveal other, more dominant, EEG abnormalities.

Spikes, sharp waves, and slow waves may arise from the partially functional neurons adjacent to the lesion. This adjacent tissue may be inflamed or degenerative. It may also be healthy, with function made abnormal by the changed equilibrium of synaptic relations with damaged neurons.

Electric activity is greatly influenced by whether the principal lesion is expanding, static, or resolving. Common causes of expanding lesions are infections, tumors, hematomas, and parasitic cysts.

The EEG is not the precise and sensitive indicator of disease that some wishfully expect it to be, but some conclusions may be tentatively drawn about certain types of EEG abnormalities.

Spikes and sharp waves presumably reflect an irritative process and occur in acute and chronic disease in which lesions are expanding. Spikes are associated with hyperirritability in humans (Hill and Parr, 1963) and are conspicuous in epileptiform activity. They may result from localized implantation of bacteriologically contaminated electrodes (Ruckebush, 1965). They may occur in diseases known to be inflammatory. In early encephalitis, for example, spikes occur in the EEG of unanesthetized dogs (Redding, 1965; Redding *et al.*, 1966). Anesthetized dogs that exhibited spikes or sharp waves (Fig. 7-10) were found at necropsy to have either perivascular cuffing or scattered necrotic neurons. Also, several dogs that recovered from bacterial encephalitis had spikes in their EEG.

Spiking does not necessarily indicate that the disease occurred recently. Subcortical cryogenic lesions in cats produce spike foci that often lasted weeks and months (Proctor *et al.*, 1966). In a study of anesthetized dogs spikes occurred in 12 dogs, 8 of which had long-standing disease, with initial signs appearing 1 month to 4 years before EEG examination (Klemm, 1968b). Spikes may indicate that a disease, if not recent, is an old condition in which there is persistent irritation of some neurons.

HVFA (Fig. 7-11) is often the major component of epileptiform activity, which some evidence indicates is an irritative process, accompanied at the cell level by much EPSP activity and diminished IPSP activity (Chapter 1, Section I, C, and Chapter 7, Section II, D).

HVSA (Fig. 7-12) is apparently the most common abnormality, as suggested by the various published reports. HVSA is not indicative of a specific abnormality, and it occurs in a wide variety of disease conditions. It may represent a later stage of disease where necrosis has begun. This is indicated by reports in unanesthetized dogs that late encephalitis is

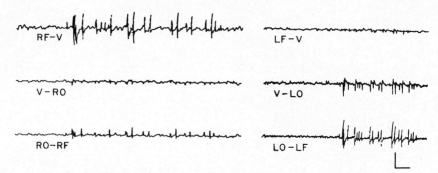

Fig. 7-10.   Localized spiking and LVFA. Bipolar phase inversion indicates that spikes originate in the right occipital (RO; left-hand traces) and the left occipital (LO; right-hand traces) regions. Recordings obtained from an anesthetized 5-year-old male Brittany spaniel that had perivascular cuffing and distemper inclusion bodies in the occipital regions. RF = right frontal; LF = left frontal; V = vertex. Calibrations: 50 μV; 1 sec. (Klemm, 1968b.)

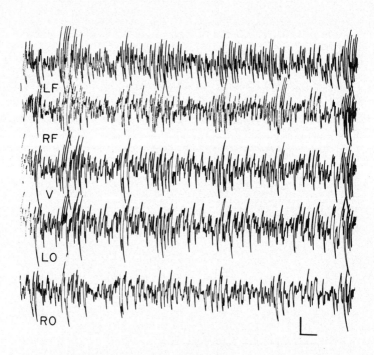

Fig. 7-11.   Conspicuous HVFA and exaggerated spindles in an anesthetized 2-year-old male toy poodle for which no diagnosis could be achieved. Abbreviations are the same as in Fig. 7-10. Calibrations: 50 μV; 1 sec. (Klemm, 1968b.)

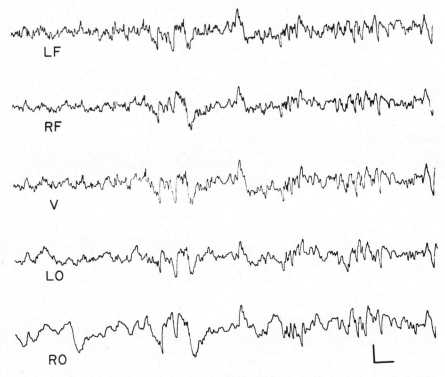

FIG. 7-12. Generalized HVSA of 1–2/sec. obtained from an anesthetized 2-year-old crossbred terrier with bilateral malacia in midbrain, cerebellum, and occipital cortex. Abbreviations are the same as in Fig. 7-10. Calibrations: 50 μV; 1 sec. (Klemm, 1968b.)

characterized by HVSA, whereas early encephalitis is not (Redding, 1965; Redding *et al.*, 1966).

Cases with excessive HVSA during anesthesia are reported to include dogs with advanced encephalitis, necrosis, malacia, subarachnoid hemorrhage, tumors, trauma, hydrocephalus, and 2 dogs in which lesions were not found (Klemm, 1968b).

Although HVSA seems to have little value in diagnosing a specific disease, it may indicate that a disease, of whatever origin, has progressed beyond the initial irritative stage. In one study (Klemm, 1968b) all of the animals with HVSA had signs of at least 4 days' duration prior to EEG examination. The 2 dogs with a 4-day history had localized HVSA, and most of the others had symptoms for weeks or months before the EEG was made.

LVFA (Fig. 7-13), like spikes, may reflect an early, irritative process. In man, such abnormality is associated with hyperexcitability (Hill and

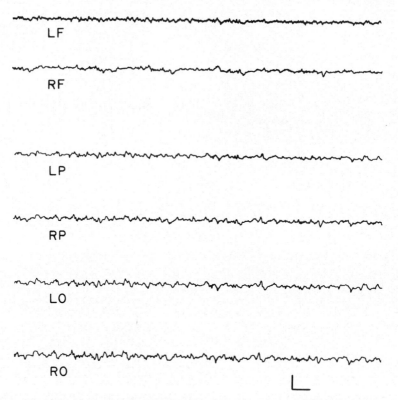

Fig. 7-13. Generalized LVFA, recorded from an anesthetized 2-year-old male St. Bernard that had had a heat stroke 7 days before. Much activity in the last 4 channels is not abnormally fast, but the voltages are low. Congested pial vessels and severe and extensive chronic pneumonia were seen at necropsy. Abbreviations are the same as in Fig. 7-10; LP and RP = left and right parietal. Calibrations: 50 μV; 1 sec. (Klemm, 1968b.)

Parr, 1963). In one study of dogs a wide range of symptoms occurred, and 3 of the 6 dogs with generalized LVFA were not hyperirritable. There was inflammatory disease in the dogs with confirmed diagnoses: heat stroke, bacterial encephalitis, toxoplasmosis,[7] and distemper (Klemm, 1968b). In unanesthetized dogs, LVFA has been attributed to early encephalitis and meningitis (Croft, 1965a,b).

There is some indication that LVFA indicates recent disease, because the symptoms usually appeared in one study less than 2 weeks prior to EEG examination. However, 2 dogs with LVFA had symptoms 6 months and 1 year before EEG examination. These findings may be consistent with those previously mentioned, if a focal inflammatory process had been recently activated (Klemm, 1968b).

[7]This dog, and 2 other unanesthetized dogs with toxoplasmosis (Redding et al., 1966), shared a common EEG finding of low voltage activity.

Occurrence of LVFA in anesthetized animals seems paradoxical, because light anesthesia normally produces a distinct shift toward HVSA. A similar paradox of LVFA has been reported in humans who were comatose because of brainstem lesions (reviewed by Otomo, 1966).

Spindle asymmetry or exaggeration seems to be abnormal. In normal, anesthetized dogs, EEG spindles are transient bursts of 6–12 sharp waves with a frequency of 6–12 sec and an incidence of about 4–9 bursts/min. The spindles are most conspicuous in records obtained by reference recording, and they are more prominent rostrally. They always appear in frontal leads and sometimes appear in all leads. Spindles within a given hemisphere had similar appearances; between hemispheres they differed slightly but did occur at approximately the same time. Spindles were of 2 basic types: one a relatively high-amplitude distinct form (similar to that illustrated in Figs. 6-1, 6-10, 6-11A, and 6-17) and the other a masked form in which spindles consisted of a low-voltage "ripple" superimposed on background activity (Fig. 7-14) (Klemm, 1968a).

Dogs with brain disease often exhibit spindle asymmetry (Fig. 7-15) or exaggeration of spindle amplitude and incidence (Fig. 7-16; Klemm, 1968b). Spindle asymmetry in sleeping humans has been associated with vascular lesions (Rohmer *et al.*, 1952). Necropsies of dogs with EEGs demonstrating spindle asymmetry revealed neuronal necrosis and bacterial and viral encephalitis (Klemm, 1968b). Exaggeration of spindles in that study occurred in 1 dog with cortical perivascular cuffing. In humans, exaggerated spindles have been reported in the sleep EEG of mentally retarded children under the age of 12 (E. L. Gibbs and Gibbs, 1962). A fast and spikey type of spindle also has been reported in children with various forms of brain disease (Niedermeyer and Capute, 1967).

Distribution of EEG abnormalities bears on diagnosis and prognosis. Certain general principles can be stated that assist in diagnosis. After abnormality is detected and classified, the major question concerns whether that abnormality is focal or diffuse. It seems reasonable to expect that *focal abnormalities indicate a focal lesion in the cortex, whereas diffuse EEG abnormalities indicate either diffuse cortical or subcortical lesions or focal subcortical lesions.* These postulates arise from volume conductor properties of the brain, wherein aberrant potentials are reflected in 3 dimensions. Subcortical brain areas have many projection paths to widespread areas of the cortex. Subcortical lesions, even if focal, should appear at several electrodes at the head's surface. Necropsy examination of animals with EEG focal and diffuse abnormalities have tended to support these ideas (Klemm, 1968b; Gastaut and Fischer-Williams, 1959; Kriendler, 1965).

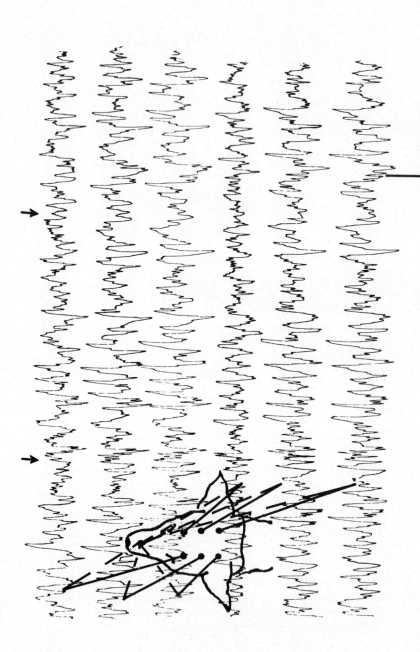

FIG. 7-14.   Appearance of presumed spindles in their "masked" form (arrows), as recorded from a normal, anesthetized dog. Spindles appear as a low voltage "ripple" superimposed on background activity. The designation of this phenomenon as "spindles" is based on observations that they occur in bursts, are sharp waves of duration like that in spindles, occur at regular intervals, and occur only in normal dogs that do not have "typical" spindles. Calibrations: 20 μV; 1 sec.

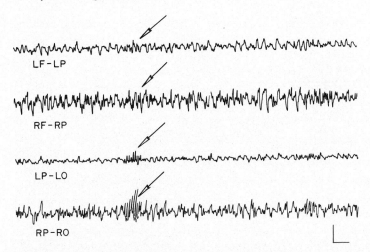

FIG. 7-15. Asymmetrical spindles (arrows), with normal spindling only in the RP-RO bipolar lead (incidence = 6–7/min). Frontal-parietal HVSA and overall asymmetry also exist. EEG was taken from an anesthetized 4-month-old male coon hound with staphylococcus encephalitis. Abbreviations are the same as in Fig. 7-13. Calibrations: 50 μV; 1 sec.

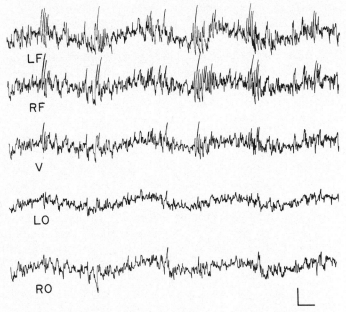

FIG. 7-16. Exaggerated spindles of high amplitude and incidence (14/min). The EEG contains some frontal HVSA of 2½–3/sec, usually in association with spindles. Records were taken from an anesthetized 8½-year-old male Boston terrier with mild, diffuse, perivascular cuffing of undetermined etiology in all of the cortex. Abbreviations are the same as in Fig. 7-10. Calibrations: 50 μV; 1 sec.

There are several exceptions to the idea that a local cortical lesion will cause only focal EEG abnormality. These include the fact that focal abnormality spreads during a seizure to activate normal neurons into abnormal firing patterns. During interictal periods a focus may trigger a "mirror" focus in contralateral homotopic cortex.

Distribution of lesions also aids in prognosis. A localized cortical lesion offers more hope for recovery than multiple cortical lesions or subcortical lesions. Subcortical lesions tend to be more dangerous to the life of the animal, and the degree of danger varies with which subcortical nuclei are affected.

Surface electroencephalography does not readily identify the origin of subcortical foci, but it may correlate significantly with clinical symptoms. The most definitive method for localizing subcortical lesions is to employ depth electrodes, a procedure that is sometimes used clinically in humans (Ramey and O'Doherty, 1960) and that may become more widely used in animals.

Distribution of EEG abnormalities also gives some hint as to the cause of the disease. *Focal EEG abnormalities suggest a disease that causes limited pathology, such as a tumor, infarct, hemorrhage, or focal necrosis. Diffuse EEG abnormalities suggest diseases such as infections, trauma, and large space-occupying lesions (tumor and hydrocephalus), which could be expected to produce widespread pathology.*

The EEG also can be valuable in prognosis. A lesion that is localized suggests a more favorable prognosis than one that is generalized. Tumors and other progressive diseases of course should be excluded. Serial recordings indicate whether the disease is progressing, thus providing better grounds for an accurate prognosis.

In one study (Klemm, 1968b) 68% accuracy on prognosis was achieved by employing the following assumptions: (1) Generalized abnormalities in the EEG may indicate widespread cortical damage or subcortical damage (focal or widespread), both of which would mitigate against a favorable prognosis. Based on the case history and symptoms, a prognosis of no major change, some deterioration, or considerable deterioration-to-death was given. (2) Localized EEG abnormalities may indicate a cortical lesion that probably would not progress and thus result in a prognosis of no major change, some improvement, or recovery (tumors excepted). (3) Generalized HVSA may indicate severe damage of many neurons from a variety of causes; depending on the history, symptoms, distribution, and severity of HVSA, the prognosis was no major change, some deterioration, or considerable deterioration to death. (4) Generalized sharp waves, spikes, and LVFA may indicate an irritative process that will likely progress, since infectious encephalitis is a common cause of these EEG abnormalities in animals. The prognosis was thus some deterioration or considerable deterioration to death.

As more knowledge is gained, better guidelines for prognosis will evolve.

D. EEG CORRELATES OF SPECIFIC DISEASES

1. Nutritional Deficiencies

EEG manifestations of nutritional disease have been reviewed by Dawson and Greville (1963). *Thiamine* (vitamin B_1) deficiency, for example, causes an initial high-voltage pattern that progressively develops into HVSA. *Pyridoxine* (vitamin B_6) deficiency causes EEG seizures, with interictal EEGs not distinctly abnormal. *Cobalamine* (vitamin B_{12}) deficiency tends to produce slowing in EEG frequencies. *Protein* deficiency produces HVSA. Overconsumption of phenylalanine induces in monkeys the disease phenylketonuria, associated with seizures and interictal EEGs of the HVSA type (Cadell *et al.*, 1962).

2. Toxins

The effects of toxins on the EEG have been reviewed by Dawson and Greville (1963). *Lead* poisoning of cats causes initial low-voltage activity of variable frequency followed by HVSA. *Sodium fluoride* tends to flatten the EEG of cats. *Cyanide* induces HVSA in the mammals that have been studied. *Methylene blue*, in *encéphalé isolé* cats, induces HVFA. *Fluoroacetate* induces epileptiform activity in dogs.

3. Irradiation

EEG effects of irradiation have been reviewed by Kimeldorf and Hunt (1965). It is difficult to generalize about the effects because quite variable responses have been reported. The inconsistencies are due in large measure to differences in species, irradiation parameters, and recording conditions. Such variation was noted in my own studies of this subject, using the same species and recording conditions (Fig. 7-17; Klemm and Bachofer, 1965).

It is clear that sublethal doses of irradiation produce EEG changes in a wide variety of species. After lethal doses, as animals become moribund, both HVSA and LVFA have been reported.

Very large doses (2–10 kr) definitely depress neural activity, accompanied by slow EEG frequencies (either high or low voltage). During

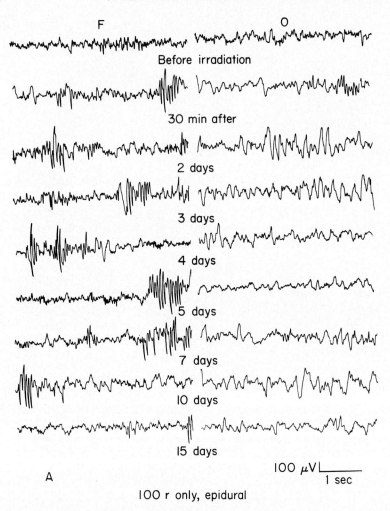

F   O

Before irradiation

30 min after

2 days

3 days

4 days

5 days

7 days

10 days

15 days

A

100 μV

1 sec

100 r only, epidural

FIG. 7-17. Effect of 2 dose levels of irradiation (x-ray) on the frontal (F) and occipital (O) EEG of rabbits. A: After 100 r, spindle incidence increases and HVSA dominates during the first 4 days. After 5 days there is less HVSA, but the spindle incidence is still high. Some indication of recovery is noted in the record at day 15. B: After 400 r there was a transient period of HVSA and spindle increase, but during days 2–5 only the spindle increase persisted. After 7 days, HVSA returned and the spindle incidence remained high.

the postirradiation period, a stage of temporary recovery and near-normal EEGs may occur.

Irradiation also can produce initial excitatory effects, associated with LVFA, which may be followed by recovery or death, depending on the dose. Many such studies, especially those by Russians, have suggested that arousal responses occur to extremely low doses (even less than 1 r). The detection and subsequent EEG reaction may be due to the sensi-

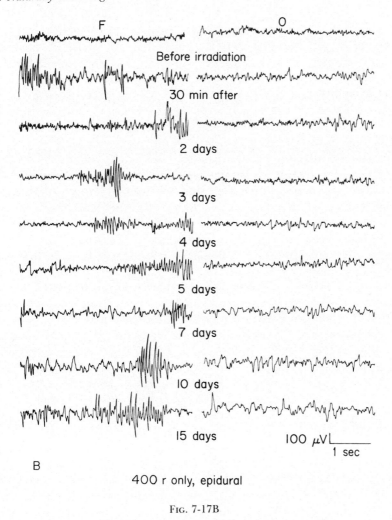

F   O

Before irradiation

30 min after

2 days

3 days

4 days

5 days

7 days

IO days

I5 days

100 μV

1 sec

B

400 r only, epidural

FIG. 7-17B

tivity of olfactory bulbs, as suggested by studies in which the EEG response was lost following removal of olfactory bulbs.

Most of the remaining discussion in this section applies to dogs. Few cats have been studied by anyone, but the 21 examined by Croft (1965a) appeared to present the same EEG abnormalities as dogs.

4. Encephalitis–Meningitis

Infectious encephalitis can cause various EEG abnormalities, with HVSA becoming especially prominent as the disease progresses.

Redding *et al.* (1966) describe 3 EEG patterns in unanesthetized, encephalitic dogs. The first pattern, associated with early encephalitis, consists of fast, 20–30/sec activity superimposed on 3–6/sec activity. The voltage is relatively low, at 5–75 μV. Also present are paroxysmal slowing, spikes, and asynchrony between contralateral leads (Fig. 7-18). Another pattern, associated with "acute" encephalitis, consists of HVSA, with frequencies of 1–3/sec and voltages of 100–200 μV (Fig. 7-19). The third pattern, associated with "late" (recovery stage) encephalitis, consists of 4–7/sec activity, 10–75 μV, with moderate synchrony of contralateral leads (Fig. 7-20). Acute and chronic encephalitic dogs also exhibited very short arousal reactions to sensory stimulation.

EEGs from normal dogs under these recording conditions revealed a LVFA of 5–25 μV and 8–20/sec during alert wakefulness and a HVSA of 25–100 μV and 2–5/sec during sleep (Figs. 7-21 and 7-22).

Croft (1965c) reported that the EEG from unanesthetized dogs with encephalitis consisted of continuous low voltage or of slow waves combined with runs of low-voltage activity. Low-voltage records were even observed in distemper cases that had progressed to the choreic stage.

The EEG abnormalities of anesthetized encephalitic dogs appear to be classifiable as LVFA or spikes (acute encephalitis) and HVSA—late encephalitis (Fig. 7-23A and B; Klemm, 1968b). Generalized LVFA and/or generalized spiking occurred in animals with acute encephalitis. All dogs that were necropsied had encephalitic lesions, as a result of heat stroke, bacterial infection, toxoplasmosis, and distemper; some other dogs had perivascular cuffing and isolated necrotic neurons of unknown cause.

The most common EEG correlate of encephalitis in anesthetized dogs was excessive and generalized HVSA, which may reflect the fact that the disease was often well established before the animal was presented for evaluation. These dogs generally had a history of symptoms of a week or more. The EEG of certain dogs contained a mixture of HVSA and spikes (as also reported by Croft for unanesthetized dogs). This finding is interpreted to indicate that the disease, although well established, is still active and spreading within the brain. Diagnoses that have been confirmed in these cases of chronic encephalitis include bacterial infection, distemper, and some cases of necrosis and malacia of unknown cause.

Although these EEG correlates of acute and chronic encephalitis seem to be reasonably well founded, information is still inadequate. Considerable insight could be gained from experimental studies in which known organisms are inoculated into an animal and the EEG changes are correlated with the development of clinical and pathologic changes.

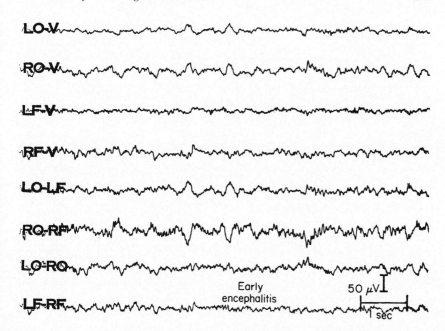

FIG. 7-18.   EEG of the early stages of viral encephalitis in the unanesthetized dog. Traces reveal a great deal of superimposed fast activity. Abbreviations are the same as in Fig. 7-10. (Redding *et al.*, 1966.)

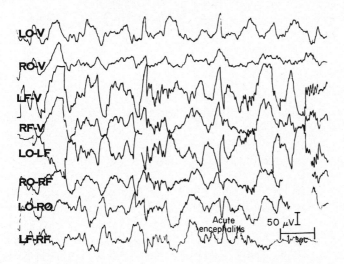

FIG. 7-19.   EEG of the more developed stages of viral encephalitis in the unanesthetized dog. Traces reveal considerable HVSA. Abbreviations are the same as in Fig. 7-10. (Redding *et al.*, 1966.)

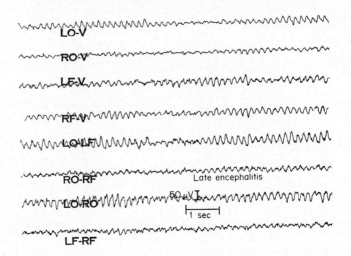

FIG. 7-20.   EEG of the late stages of viral encephalitis in the unanesthetized dog. Traces reveal 4–7/sec HVSA in the more caudal areas that is moderately synchronous in contralateral leads. Abbreviations are the same as in Fig. 7-10. (Redding *et al.*, 1966.)

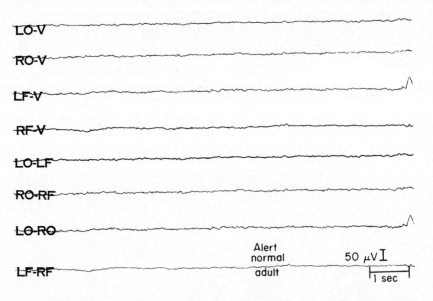

FIG. 7-21.   EEG of a normal unanesthetized dog during alert wakefulness. Traces reveal LVFA of about 8–20/sec and 5–25 μV. Abbreviations are the same as in Fig. 7-10. (Redding *et al.*, 1966.)

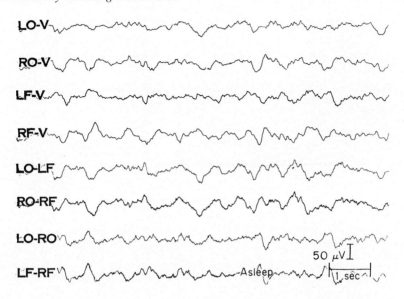

FIG. 7-22. EEG of a normal unanesthetized dog during natural sleep. Traces reveal HVSA of about 3-5/sec. along with superimposed faster activity. Abbreviations are the same as in Fig. 7-10. (Redding *et al.*, 1966.)

Unfortunately, not many such studies have been performed. In one study (Griffith *et al.*, 1967) herpes simplex virus inoculation into rabbits caused death in 4 of 6 in 6-20 days. The 2 surviving rabbits revealed no EEG abnormalities nor conspicuous clinical symptoms. The 4 sick rabbits all revealed EEG abnormalities of spikes and sharp waves prior to the onset of clinical symptoms. Some of the sharp waves were clustered in bursts, appearing as exaggerated spindles. As the disease progressed to preterminal stages, sharp waves were largely replaced with HVSA or slow waves of low voltage.

5. Vascular Disorders

Either infarcts or hemorrhages would be expected to produce abnormal EEGs. However, few naturally occurring cases with EEG studies have been reported. Two investigators reported 1-2/sec HVSA in connection with subdural hematomas (Fig. 7-24; Redding *et al.*, 1966; Redding, 1965; Croft, 1963). HVSA of 1-2/sec was also reported in an anesthetized dog with subarachnoid hemorrhage (Klemm, 1968b).

Vascular disorders would be expected to produce anoxia and, as discussed in Chapter 6, Section III, A, would probably result in HVSA,

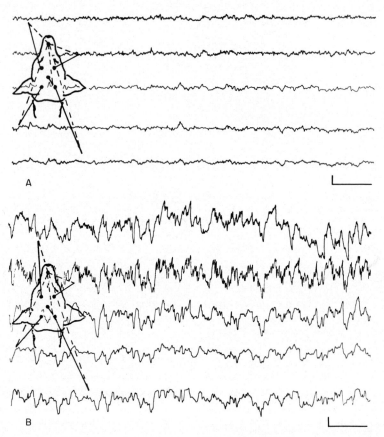

FIG. 7-23.   A: EEG from an anesthetized, 5-year-old dog with acute encephalitis, later diagnosed at necropsy as due to distemper. There were no gross lesions, only perivascular cuffing and intranuclear inclusions in astroglial cells of the cortex. Calibrations: 20 μV; 1 sec. B: EEG from an anesthetized, adult terrier crossbred with chronic encephalitis. Dog had been developing symptoms of distemper for several weeks and at the time of EEG recording had pronounced chorea of the head and left leg and was unable to stand. Necropsy revealed necrosis and malacia, along with enlarged astrocytes with intranuclear inclusions and only a mild degree of perivascular cuffing in the cortex. Calibrations: 20 μV; 2 sec.

the distribution of which would depend on the anatomy of the affected vasculature. For example, I observed that an adult German shepherd with focal HVSA had focal cortical hemorrhage, whereas an adult cross bred with generalized HVSA had hemorrhage around the brainstem.

A fairly common cause of brain anoxia is anesthetic accident in which the heart stops beating during surgery. If circulation cannot be restored

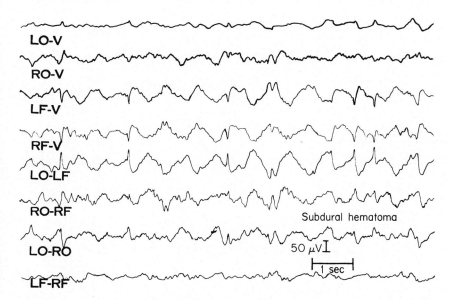

LO-V

RO-V

LF-V

RF-V

LO-LF

RO-RF

Subdural hematoma

LO-RO

50 μV

1 sec

LF-RF

FIG. 7-24. EEG of an unanesthetized dog suffering from a subdural hematoma. Traces reveal 1–2/sec HVSA, with focus especially apparent over the left frontal region. Abbreviations are the same as in Fig. 7-10. (Redding, 1965.)

within about 5 min, permanent brain damage will result. The EEG of a cat in which prolonged cardiac arrest occurred is shown in Fig. 7-25. The EEG was taken 2 months after the accident, and it reveals a peculiar pattern of HVSA and sharp waves. The occipital activity was identical, and this was used to illustrate bipolar cancellation effects in Fig. 5-5. Clinically, the cat was blind and spent most of the time staring blankly upward.

Naquet *et al.* (1966) injected air into the carotid arteries of cats in order to produce and study gas embolism. Such treatment produced an initial, transient, generalized isoelectric EEG over the affected hemisphere. After a variable period of HVSA, near normal EEGs returned, but in about half the cases, at about the sixth hour, paroxysmal spikes and sharp waves occurred which disappeared between the twenty-fourth and thirty-sixth hour.

6. Trauma

Trauma is very often associated with vascular lesions, and the previous comments would seem applicable here. However, trauma can cause damage independently of vascular lesions. Concussion is reported to cause an initial flattening of the EEG, followed within a few hours by generalized HVSA (Redding, 1965).

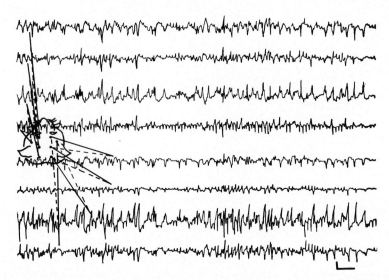

Fig. 7-25.   EEG from an anesthetized cat that had experienced cardiac arrest 2 months earlier. Sharp waves and HVSA are prominent; definite foci appear to exist in temporal and occipital regions. Calibrations: 20 μV; 1 sec.

I have studied 4 cases of trauma, resulting from car accidents or falling down stairs, in which the EEG during anesthesia consisted of generalized HVSA (Fig. 7-26).

7. Hydrocephalus

Two investigators (Croft, 1965b; Redding, 1965) reported similar findings in cases of hydrocephalus. The EEG contained runs of 6–10/sec HVSA, with voltages ranging toward 300 μV (Fig. 7-27A). However, the predominant EEG abnormality in the 3 hydrocephalus cases reported by deLahunta and Cummings (1965) was generalized 1–3/sec HVSA. Similarly, the 8 confirmed cases of Prynn and Redding (1968) had a predominance of 1–5/sec HVSA, with some records also revealing a superimposed 6–20/sec activity. The anesthetized case I have seen (Fig. 7-27B) also revealed extreme 0.5–5/sec voltages; superimposed 6–10/sec activity was present in some traces, and there were definite differences in activity between hemispheres. Although generalized HVSA appears to be a consistent accompaniment of hydrocephalus,[8] this type of EEG abnormality can occur with other disease conditions, such as tumors and trauma.

[8]Prynn reports in a personal communication (1968) having observed a flat EEG in a case of hydrocephalus.

8. Tumors

Tumors are reported to produce HVSA (Croft, 1963, 1965b; Redding, 1965), and this is consistent with the findings from the several anesthetized tumor cases I have seen. The distribution of EEG abnormality depends on the location of the tumor. If the tumor is deep and remote from electrodes, abnormalities may be minimal or, if present, will be present at several electrode sites. More superficial tumors can cause very pronounced HVSA; even though the tumor tissue itself may be electrically silent, the pressure on adjacent tissue causes considerable disruption of function.

9. Conclusions

The discussion on specific diseases should emphasize the limits of our present knowledge. Veterinary electroencephalography is a relatively new specialty, and we can reasonably expect great progress in the future. Progress will be accelerated by more EEG studies of experimentally produced brain lesions that simulate the naturally occurring diseases. Use of specialized techniques, such as depth electrography and evoked response analysis, should also be of great benefit.

Present knowledge indicates that the EEG, by itself, does not facilitate *differential* diagnosis. However, when evaluated with reference to clinical history, symptoms, and other diagnostic tests, the EEG can be a very important tool in differential diagnosis. Regarding indications of

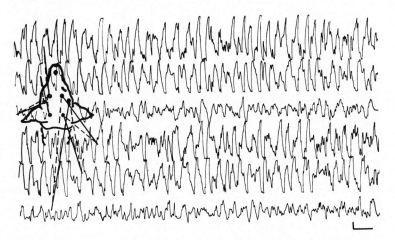

FIG. 7-26. EEG from an anesthetized, 3-month-old puppy that had been hit by a car 2 days earlier. The dog was ataxic and having convulsions prior to anesthesia. Tracings reveal marked HVSA and foci of abnormality especially prominent over occipital regions. Calibrations: 20 μV: 1 sec.

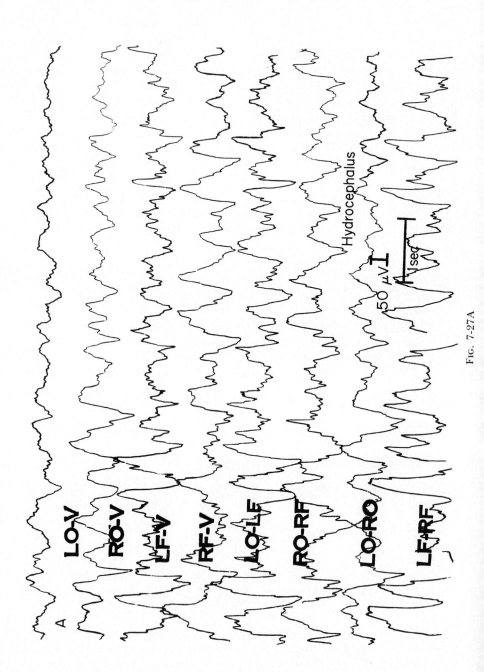

Fɪɢ. 7-27A

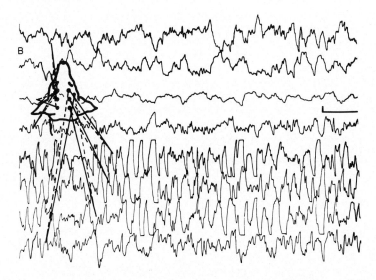

FIG. 7-27. A: EEG from an unanesthetized dog with hydrocephalus. Traces reveal 1–2/sec HVSA. Abbreviations are the same as in Fig. 7-10. (Pyrnn and Redding, 1968.) B: EEG from an anesthetized, 12-week-old Dachsund with hydrocephalus. Runs of 6–10/sec are evident in some traces (left temporal–left frontal), but the dominant feature is extremely high-voltage 1–4/sec activity. Foci of abnormality are especially prominent at left frontal, left central, right central, and right occipital. Activity in the right hemisphere is conspicuously different from that in the left. Calibrations: 50 μV; 1 sec.

specific diseases, present understanding permits only an estimation of the type of predominant disease process, as either inflammatory or degenerative. Although evidence is inconclusive, it may be that inflammatory diseases (acute infection or toxins) are indicated by EEG LVFA, spikes, or sharp waves. Degenerative disease may be indicated by HVSA (chronic infection, trauma, tumors, hydrocephalus, or vascular disorders).

At present there do seem to be grounds for concluding that the EEG can be successfully used to determine (1) if there is brain disease, (2) the distribution of lesions, (3) the severity of lesions, (4) the character of the lesion's cause (inflammation or degeneration), and (5) prognosis of the disease outcome.

REFERENCES

Ajmone Marsan, C. (1965). Micro-structural mechanisms of seizure susceptibility. *Excerpta Med. Found., Intern. Congr. Ser.* **124**, 47–59.

Ajmone Marsan, C. (1966). Epilepsy. *Progr. Neurol. Psychiat.* **21**, 195–260.

Cadell, T. E., Harlow, H. F., and Waisman, H. A. (1962). EEG changes in experimental phenylketonuria. *Electroencephalog. Clin. Neurophysiol.* **14**, 540–543.

Chow, K. L., and Obrist, W. D. (1954). EEG changes on application of Al(OH)$_3$ cream on the cortex. *A.M.A. Arch. Neurol. Psychiat.* **72**, 80–87.

Coceani, F., Libman, I., and Gloor, P. (1966). The effect of intracorotid amobarbital injections upon experimentally induced epileptiform activity. *Electroencephalog. Clin. Neurophysiol.* **20**, 542–558.

Croft, P. G. (1963). The EEG as an aid to diagnosis of nervous diseases in the dog and cat. *J. Small Animal Pract.* **3**, 205–213.

Croft, P. G. (1965a). Conditions affecting the central nervous system in small animals. *J. Small Animal Pract.* **6**, 261–271.

Croft, P. G. (1965b). Use of the electroencephalogram in small animal medicine. *Proc. Roy. Soc. Med.* **58**, 548–549.

Croft, P. G. (1965c). Fits in dogs: A survey of 260 cases. *Vet. Record* **77**, 438–445.

Dawson, M. E., and Greville, G. D. (1963). Biochemistry. *In* "Electroencephalography" (D. Hill and G. Parr, eds.), pp. 147–192. Macmillan, New York.

deLahunta, A., and Cummings, J. F. (1965). The clinical and electroencephalographic features of hydrocephalus in three dogs. *J. Am. Vet. Med. Assoc.* **146**, 954–964.

Dow, R. S., Fernández-Guardiola, A., and Manni, E. (1962). The production of cobalt experimental epilepsy in the rat. *Electroencephalog. Clin. Neurophysiol.* **14**, 399–407.

Feher, O., Halasz, P., and Mechler, F. (1965). The mechanism of or origin of cortical convulsive potentials. *Electroencephalog. Clin. Neurophysiol.* **19**, 541–548.

Frank, G. S., Fraser, R. A. R., and Whitcher, C. (1966). Intramuscular methohexital for rapid induction of short duration sleep in the EEG laboratory: A study of forty-four hyperkinetic children. *Electroencephalog. Clin. Neurophysiol.* **21**, 76–78.

Gastaut, H., and Fischer-Williams, M. (1959). The physiopathology of epileptic seizures. *In* "Handbook of Physiology" (Am. Physiol. Soc., J. Field, ed.), Sect. 1, Vol. I, pp. 329–363. Williams & Wilkins, Baltimore, Maryland.

Gibbs, E. L., and Gibbs, F. A. (1962). Extreme spindles: Correlation of electroencephalographic sleep patterns with mental retardation. *Science* **138**, 1106.

Gibbs, F. A., and Gibbs, E. L. (1965). "Medical Electroencephalography." Addison-Wesley, Reading, Massachusetts.

Gibbs, F. A., Gibbs, E. L., and Fuster, B. (1947). Anterior temporal localization of sleep-induced seizure discharges of the psychomotor type. *Trans. Am. Neurol. Assoc.* 180–182.

Goodman, S. J., and Mann, P. E. G. (1967). Reticular and thalamic multiple unit activity during wakefulness, sleep, and anesthesia. *Exptl. Neurol.* **19**, 11–24.

Griffith, J. F., Kibrick, S., Dodge, P. R., and Richardson, E. P. (1967). Experimental herpes simplex encephalitis. *Electroencephalog. Clin. Neurophysiol.* **23**, 263–269.

Herin, R. A., Purinton, P. T., and Fletcher, T. F. (1968). Electroencephalography in the unanesthetized dog. *Am. J. Vet. Res.* **29**, 329–336.

Hill, D., and Parr, G. eds. (1963). "Electroencephalography." Macmillan, New York.

Hoerlein, B. F. (1965). "Canine Neurology." Saunders, Philadelphia, Pennsylvania.

Kimeldorf, D. J., and Hunt, E. L. (1965). "Ionizing Radiation." Academic Press, New York.

Klemm, W. R. (1968a). Subjective and quantitative analyses of the electroencephalogram of anesthetized normal dogs — control data for clinical diagnosis. *Am. J. Vet. Res.* **29**, 1267–1277.

Klemm, W. R. (1968b). Electroencephalograms of anesthetized dogs and cats with neurologic diseases. *Am. J. Vet. Res.* **29**, 337–351.

Klemm, W. R. (1968c). Attempts to standardize veterinary electroencephalographic techniques. *Am. J. Vet. Res.* **29**, 1895–1900.

Klemm, W. R., and Bachofer, C. S. (1965). Psychotropic drug and adrenal-pituitary influences on radiation-induced changes in brain electrical activity and behavior. *Radiation Res.* **24**, 201–213.

Klemm, W. R., and Mallo, G. L. (1966). Clinical electroencephalography in anesthetized small animals. *J. Am. Vet. Med. Assoc.* **148**, 1038–1042.

Kogi, K., Nakamura, Y., Miyama, T., and Kawamura, H. (1960). Effect of ethyl alcohol on electrical activity of neo-, paleo-, and archicortical systems. *Rept. Inst. Sci. Labour* **56**, 1–14.

Kriendler, A. (1965). Experimental Epilepsy. *Progr. Brain. Res.* **19**.

McGrath, J. T. (1960). "Neurologic Examination of the Dog." Lea & Febiger, Philadelphia, Pennsylvania.

Matsumoto, H. (1964). Intracellular events during the activation of cortical epileptiform discharges. *Electroencephalog. Clin. Neurophysiol.* **17**, 294–307.

Matsumoto, H., and Ajmone Marsan, C. (1964). Cellular mechanisms in experimental epileptic seizures. *Science* **144**, 193–194.

Monnier, M., and Gangloff, H. (1961). "Atlas for Stereotoxic Brain Research on the Conscious Rabbit." Elsevier, Amsterdam.

Morillo, A., and Baylor, D. (1964). A brief report on the experimental production of electroclinical patterns of petit mal type. *Electroencephalog. Clin. Neurophysiol.* **16**, 519–521.

Nakamura, Y., and Ohye, C. (1964). Delta wave production in neocortical EEG by acute lesions within thalamus and hypothalamus of the cat. *Electroencephalog. Clin. Neurophysiol.* **17**, 677–684.

Naquet, R., Arfel, G., Choux, M., Dubois, D., and Riche, D. (1966). Etude expérimentale di l'embolie gazeuse par voie carotidienne chez le chat. *Electroencephalog. Clin. Neurophysiol.* **20**, 181–196.

Niedermeyer, E., and Capute, A. J. (1967). A fast and spikey spindle variant in children with organic brain disease. *Electroencephalog. Clin. Neurophysiol.* **23**, 67–73.

Otomo, E. (1966). Beta wave activity in the electroencephalogram in cases of coma due to acute brain-stem lesions. *J. Neurol., Neurosurg., Psychiat.* **29**, 383–390.

Palmer, A. C. (1965). "Introduction to Animal Neurology." Davis, Philadelphia, Pennsylvania.

Pollen, D. A., Reid, K. H., and Perot, P. (1964). Micro-electrode studies of experimental 3/sec wave and spike in the cat. *Electroenecphalog. Clin. Neurophysiol.* **17**, 57–67.

Proctor, F., Prince, D. A., and Morrell, F. (1966). Primary and secondary spike foci following depth lesions. *Arch. Neurol.* **15**, 152–162.

Prynn, R. B. (1968). Personal communication.

Prynn, R. B., and Redding, R. W. (1968). Electroencephalogram in occult canine hydrocephalus. *J. Am. Vet. Med. Assoc.* **152**, 1651–1657.

Ramey, E. R., and O'Doherty, D. S., eds. (1960). "Electrical Studies on the Unanesthetized Brain." Harper (Hoeber), New York.

Redding, R. W. (1964). A simple technique for obtaining an electroencephalogram of the dog. *Am. J. Vet. Res.* **25**, 854–857.

Redding, R. W. (1965). Canine electroencephalography. *In* "Canine Neurology" (B. F. Hoerlein, ed.), pp. 55–70. Saunders, Philadelphia, Pennsylvania.

Redding, R. W., and Colwell, R. K. (1964). Verification of the significance of canine electroencephalogram by comparison with electrocorticogram. *Am. J. Vet. Res.* **25**, 857–860.

Redding, R. W., Prynn, B., and Wagner, J. L. (1966). Clinical use of the electroencephalogram in canine encephalitis. *J. Am. Vet. Med. Assoc.* **148**, 141–149.

Rohmer, F., Gastaut, Y., and Dell, M. B. (1952). L'EEG dans la pathologie vasculaire du cerveau. *Rev. Neurol.* **87**, 93–144.

Rovit, R. L., and Swiecicki, M. (1965). Some characteristics of multiple acute epileptogenic foci in cats. *Electroencephalog. Clin. Neurophysiol.* **18**, 608–616.

Ruckebush, Y. (1965). The normal and pathological electroencephalogram of ruminants. *Proc. Roy. Soc. Med.* **58**, 551–552.

Sadove, M. S., Becka, D., and Gibbs, F. A. (1967). "Electroencephalography for Anesthesiologists and Surgeons." J. Lippincott, Philadelphia, Pennsylvania.

Sawa, M., Kaji, S., and Usuki, K. (1965). Intracellular phenomena in electrically induced seizures. *Electroencephalog. Clin. Neurophysiol.* **19**, 248–255.

Straw, R. N., and Mitchell, C. L. (1966). A study on the duration of cortical after-discharge in the cat. *Electroencephalog. Clin. Neurophysiol.* **21**, 54–58.

Visser, S. L. (1962). The reactivity of alumina cream foci in rabbits. *Electroencephalog. Clin. Neurophysiol.* **14**, 747–750.

Proposal for an EEG Terminology by the Terminology Committee of the International Federation for Electroencephalography and Clinical Neurophysiology[1]

Before presenting the glossary some general remarks should be made. (1) From the beginning the glossary has been intended for practical general use in day-by-day clinical electroencephalography. For this reason certain terms and definitions, well known by long and general use, have not been changed, though this might have been preferable for the sake of overall consistency. For example, some Greek letters (delta, theta, and beta) are used solely to indicate frequency bands, whereas others (alpha, lambda, mu, and sigma) are used to indicate specific phenomena. (2) In principle, terms used in EEG may be regarded from different points of view and may be divided in different classes. From these, for the present purpose, the most important are the following: (a) Terms descriptive of the graphic components of the EEG, irrespective of the subject's condition. For example: delta waves, spikes, etc. may be distinguished and measured without further information. (b) Terms related to certain biologic phenomena. For example: the alpha rhythm has certain EEG aspects (frequency, topography, etc.) and certain biologic aspects (eyes shut, relaxation, etc.) (3) The terms and definitions of the glossary are mainly those necessary for the description of the primary EEG as recorded directly from the scalp. (4) All EEG phenomena should be described, so far as possible, in terms of frequency or period, amplitude, phase relations, morphology, topography, quantity, and reactivity and the variability of these parameters. (5) Eponymous terminology is not accepted, following the example set by Berger, who rejected the use of his name for "alpha rhythm." (6) Greek letters should not be used as substantives, only as adjectives; thus: delta waves, delta rhythm, etc., but never "deltas." (7) Various terms and definitions are

[1]W. Storm van Leeuwen (Chairman), R. Bickford, M. Brazier (*ex officio*), W. A. Cobb, M. Dondey, H. Gastaut, P. Gloor, C. E. Henry, R. Hess, J. R. Knott, J. Kugler, G. C. Lairy, C. Loeb, O. Magnus, L. Oller Daurella, H. Petsche, R. Schwab, W. G. Walter, and L. Widen; reprinted by permission of *Electroenceph. Clin. Neurophysiol.* **20**: 293–320, 1966.

still under discussion. Moreover, changes and additions may be necessary. For this reason it is recommended that a new terminology committee be formed and that one of its tasks be an investigation into the actual use of the terms. (8) Some terms have been included without definition because their use in EEG is as in more general usage (for example, artifact) or because the components have been defined (for example, slow-wave complex).

Glossary

Abundance: use of this term has been rejected in favor of "quantity"

Activity: any sequence of waves

Alpha: used to indicate a specific phenomenon (see alpha rhythm)

Alpha equivalent: use discouraged because there is no need for the term

Alpha rhythm: rhythm, usually with frequency of 8–13 cps in adults, most prominent in the posterior areas, present most markedly when the eyes are closed, and attenuated during attention, especially visual

Alpha wave: an individual component of an alpha rhythm.

Alphoid rhythm: use discouraged because it has no relation to the alpha rhythm apart from its frequency

Artifact:

Attenuation: decrease in amplitude of activity

Background activity: more or less general and continuous activity, in contrast with paroxysmal and focal activities. Comment: Not synonymous with alpha rhythm. The need of the term is felt when referring to activity other than the one under discussion. For example, when describing a spike, it may be convenient to refer to other EEG activity as "background activity"

Beta: used to indicate a frequency band, that is, frequencies higher than 13 cps

Beta rhythm: rhythm with frequency higher than 13 cps

Beta wave: wave with a duration of less than 1/13 sec and usually forming part of a beta rhythm

Bilateral: occurring on both sides of the head

Blocking of (alpha rhythm): the use of this term is discouraged because it implies unwarranted physiologic assumptions; instead use "attenuation"

Burst: see "Paroxysm"

Common reference lead: lead that is the same in all derivations of a montage. Comment: Abbreviated "common reference" (R). See also "Montage"

Common average reference lead: the common lead is the average of potential differences at a number of electrodes. Replaces "Goldmann." See also "Montage"

Complex: group of two or more waves, clearly distinguished from background activity and occurring with a well-recognized form or recurring with consistent form. Example: "Spike and wave complex"

Cycle: the complete series of potential changes undergone by a wave before the same series is repeated

Delta: used to indicate a frequency band or a period, that is, frequency of less than 4 cps and a period of more than ¼ sec

Delta activity: series of regular or irregular waves with durations of more than ¼ sec

Delta rhythm: rhythm with frequency of less than 4 cps

Delta wave: wave with a duration of more than ¼ sec

Delta "de jeunesse" and pathological delta: the use of these terms is discouraged because of the mixture of clinical and descriptive EEG terms and the unwarranted conclusions as to age and pathology

Depth EEG: EEG derived from electrodes in direct contact with subcortical structures

Derivation: recording from a pair of leads See also: "Montage"

Diffuse: occurring over large areas without constant location; used to describe activity occurring more or less simultaneously (without necessarily being synchronous) in large areas. (A spatial parameter; compare "Random")

Diphasic: see: "Phase"

Driving: occurrence of waves phase-locked with rhythmic stimuli. Comment: If rhythmic waves occurring during rhythmic stimulation have no constant phase relations to the stimuli, the reaction should not be called driving

Duration of a wave: time interval from beginning to end of a wave. Comment: The duration of a cycle is called "Period"

Dysrhythmia: the use of this term is discouraged because widely differing meanings are attached to it by different authors and no agreement can be obtained on any one of them

Electrocorticogram (ECoG): record of electric activity derived from electrodes in direct contact with the cortex

Electroencephalogram (EEG): record of electric activity of the brain

Electric silence: absence of electric activity

Episode:

Focus: a limited region involved by, or the point of maximum potential of, a specified wave or activity (for example, spike focus, slow-wave focus)

Frequency: the number of complete cycles of a rhythm in 1 sec

Gamma: the use of this term is discouraged as it serves no useful purpose

Ground rhythm: the use of this term is discouraged; instead use "Background activity"

Harmonic:

Hypersynchrony, hypersynchronous: the use of these terms is discouraged because two or more activities may or may not be synchronous, they cannot be hypo- or hypersynchronous

Index: the percentage of time occupied by the waves specified (for example, alpha index) with larger than specified amplitude (usually 10 μV) in a given sample (usually of 1 min duration). Comment: According to the definition, waves below a given amplitude are not counted. This limitation is necessary because of noise and other factors

Intermittent delta rhythm:

Isolated slow wave:

K complex: variable combination of sharp wave, slow wave, and sigma paroxysm occurring with maximal voltage over the vertex in response to sudden stimuli, especially during sleep. Comment: The definition is not rigid as the phenome-

non shows considerable interindividual variation, though it is not difficult to recognize

Kappa wave or rhythm: the use of this term is discouraged because it serves no useful purpose

Lambda wave: sharp wave in the occipital areas, mainly positive in relation to other areas, and usually evoked by visual exploration

Lead: term used to denote a single electrode placement. See also "Montage"

Location: refers to brain areas

Low voltage EEG: EEG in which no activity larger than 20 μV can be recorded between any two points on the scalp. Comment: The value of 20 μV is arbitrary, being generally found useful

Monophasic: see "Phase"

Monopolar: the use of this term is discouraged because the term implies that it might be possible to lead from one pole only (see "Lead" and "Derivation"), which is a physical impossibility

Montage: a combination of a number of derivations. **Lead** denotes single electrode placement. **Derivation** denotes recording from a pair of leads. Comment: A montage may have a common reference lead. The common reference may be a common average reference

Morphology: the shape (form) of a wave or activity

Mu rhythm: rhythms at 7–11 cps in central region, often with arcade or comb form, associated with beta rhythm, attenuated by real, imagined, or intended movement or tactile stimulation, particularly of the hands. Comment: This is a specific term which replaces the name given originally to it, "Rythme en arceau" and names such as "Palissade," "Wicket," and "Comb" rhythm

Paroxysm: group of waves that appears and disappears abruptly and is clearly distinguished from background activity by different frequency, morphology, or amplitude. Comment: The term is not necessarily associated with pathology. Synonym: "Burst"

Period: duration of a cycle. Comment: The period is the reciprocal of the frequency of a rhythm

Petit mal variant: the use of the term is discouraged for the same reasons as given for "Delta de jeunesse"

Phase: strictly, amplitude-time relations of sinusoidal waves; loosely, time relations of different parts of a wave (or waves) in a single trace or of a wave (or waves) as recorded simultaneously in different traces. Comment: By strictly is meant in a physical sense; by loosely, as commonly used in EEG

    Monophasic: (wave) deflected to one side of the base line

    Diphasic: (wave) deflected first to one side, then to the other of the base line

    Polyphasic: (wave) deflected several times in opposite senses

Polyspike and wave: see "Spike and wave"

Positive spike:

Quantity: amount of activity in terms of amplitude and number of waves, with respect to time

Random: recurring at inconstant time intervals. Comment: "Diffuse"

Reactivity: changeability of the EEG following change in the environment

Rhythm: activity of approximately constant period and morphology, but not necessarily of amplitude

Sharp and slow wave complex: complex of two waves, one having a duration between $\frac{1}{12}$ and $\frac{1}{5}$ sec, the other between $\frac{1}{2}$ and 1 sec; this term replaces "Slow spike and wave" because "Slow spike" is thought to be a contradiction in terms (see "Sharp wave")

Sharp wave: wave distinguished from background activity with a duration of more than $\frac{1}{12}$ and less than $\frac{1}{5}$ sec. Comment: The term replaces "Slow spike" because a spike, by definition, lasts $\frac{1}{12}$ sec or less

Sigma: used to indicate a specific phenomenon (see "Sigma rhythm")

Sigma rhythm: episodic rhythm at about 14 cps usually diffuse, with a maximum near the vertex, usually occurring during certain stages of sleep. Synonym: "Sigma spindle." Comment: The term replaces "Sleep spindle"

Sigma spindle: see "Sigma rhythm"

Slow spike: the use of this term is discouraged (see "Sharp wave")

Slow wave: wave with a duration of more than $\frac{1}{8}$ sec. Comment: Slow waves, therefore, include theta and delta waves

Slow wave complex:

Spike: wave distinguished from background activity and having a duration of $\frac{1}{12}$ sec or less

Spike and wave complex: complex of two waves, one with a duration of $\frac{1}{12}$ sec or less ("Spike") and the other with a duration of $\frac{1}{5}$–$\frac{1}{2}$ sec ("Wave")

    Polyspike and wave complex: spike and wave complex with more than one spike. Synonym: "Multiple spike and wave complex"

Spike and wave rhythm: bilaterally synchronous spike and wave complexes, recurring rhythmically with a frequency of $2\frac{1}{2}$–$3\frac{1}{2}$ cps, closely associated with clinical petit mal seizures

Suppression: the use of this term is discouraged because it implies unwarranted physiologic conclusions

Theta: used to indicate a frequency band or a period, that is, frequency of 4 cps to less than 8 cps or period of $\frac{1}{4}$ sec to more than $\frac{1}{8}$ sec

Theta activity: series of regular or irregular waves with durations of $\frac{1}{4}$ to more than $\frac{1}{8}$ sec

Theta rhythm: rhythm with frequency of 4 cps to less than 8 cps

Theta wave: wave with a duration of $\frac{1}{4}$ sec to more than $\frac{1}{8}$ sec

Topography: distribution of activity with respect to anatomical landmarks. Synonym: "Spatial distribution." Comment: see "Location"

Transient: any single wave (spike, sharp wave, etc.) or brief complex, notably different from background activity

Unilateral: occurring on one side of the head

Vertex sharp wave: sharp wave, maximal at the vertex and negative in relation to other areas, often associated with arousal stimuli. Comment: Replaces "Vertex spike" because the phenomenon lasts longer than 1/12 sec

Wave: any transient change of potential difference in the EEG

List of Terms

Still under Discussion

Activation
Alpha variant rhythm
Discharge
Evoked potential and evoked response
Generalized
Hypsarrhythmia
Phase reversal
Six and fourteen per second positive spikes
Synchronization

On the basis of the above the EEG may be regarded as consisting of
1. *Waves*
   Transient
      Spike
      Sharp wave
      Vertex sharp wave
      Lambda wave
   Beta wave
   Alpha wave
   Slow wave
      Theta wave
      Delta wave
2. *Activities*
   Beta activity
   Alpha activity
   Theta activity
   Delta activity
A. *Rhythms*
   Beta rhythm
   Alpha rhythm
   Theta rhythm
   Delta rhythm
   Mu rhythm
   Sigma rhythm
   Spike and wave rhythm
B. *Complexes*
   Spike and wave complex
   Polyspike and wave complex
   K complex

So far as possible they should be described in the following parameters:
1. Frequency or period
2. Amplitude
3. Phase relations
4. Quantity
5. Morphology
6. Topography
7. Reactivity
8. Variability

Equivalent Terms

English	French	German	Italian	Spanish
Activity	Activité	Tätigkeit	Attività	Actividad
Alpha rhythm	Rhythme alpha	Alpha-Rhythmus	Ritmo alfa	Ritmo alfa
Alpha wave	Onde alpha	Alpha-Welle	Onda alfa	Onda alfa
Attenuation	Atténuation	Abflachung	Attenuazione	Atenuación
Background activity	Activitè de fond	Hintergrund-tätigkeit	Attività di fondo	Actividad de fondo
Beta rhythm	Rythme bêta	Beta-Rhythmus	Ritmo beta	Ritmo beta
Beta wave	Onde bêta	Beta-Welle	Onda beta	Onda beta
Bilateral	Bilatéral	Bilateral	Bilaterale	Bilateral
Common average reference lead	Référence commune moyenne	Sammelschiene, Mittelwert-selektrode	Referenza media	Conductor de referencia media

Equivalent Terms

English	French	German	Italian	Spanish
Common reference lead	Référence commune	Gemeinsame Bezugselektrode	Referenza comune	Conductor de referencia comun
Complex	Complexe	Komplex	Complesso	Complejo
Cycle	Cycle	Zyklus	Ciclo	Ciclo
Delta activity	Activité delta	Delta-Tätigkeit	Attività delta	Actividad delta
Delta rhythm	Rythme delta	Delta-Rhythmus	Ritmo delta	Ritmo delta
Delta wave	Onde delta	Delta-Welle	Onda delta	Onda delta
Depth EEG	EEG de profondeur	Tiefen-Elektrogramm	EEG di profondità	EEG profunda
Derivation	Dèrivation	Ableitung	Derivazione	Derivacion
Diffuse	Diffus	Diffus	Diffuso	Difuso
Diphasic	Diphasique	Biphasisch	Difasico	Difasico
Driving	Entraînement	Phasengekoppelte Reizfolgeantwort	Trascinamento	Inducción
Duration	Durée	Dauer	Durata	Duración
Electrical silence	Silence électrique	Elektrische Stille	Silenzio elettrico	Silencio electrico
Electrocorticogram (ECoG)	Electrocorticogramme	Elektrokortikogramm	Elettrocorticogramma	Electrocorticograma
Electroencephalogram (EEG)	Electroencéphalogramme	Elektroenzephalogramm	Elettroencefalogramma	Electroencefalograma
Focus	Foyer	Herd	Focolaio	Foco
Frequency	Fréquence	Frequenz	Frequenza	Frecuencia
Index	Index	Index	Indice	Indice
K complex	Complexe K	K-Komplex	Complesso K	Complejo K
Lambda wave	Onde lambda	Lambda-Welle	Onda lambda	Onda lambda
Lead	Électrode	Ableitestelle	Elettrodo	Conductor
Location	Localisation	Lokalisation	Localizzazione	Localización
Low voltage EEG	EEG de bas voltage	Flaches EEG	EEG di basso voltaggio	EEG de bajo voltaje
Monophasic	Monophasique	Monophasisch	Monofasico	Monofasico
Montage	Montage	Montage	Montaggio	Montaje
Morphology	Morphologie	Wellenform	Morfologia	Morfologia
Mu rhythm	Rythme mu	My-Rhythmus	Ritmo mu	Ritmo mi
Paroxysm	Paroxysme	Paroxysmus	Parossismo	Paroxismo
Period	Période	Wellendauer	Periodo	Periodo
Phase	Phase	Phase	Fase	Fase
Polyphasic	Polyphasique	Polyphasisch	Polifasico	Polifásica
Polyspike and wave	Poly-pointe onde	Poly-Spike-Wave	Polipunta-onda	Polipunta-onda
Random	Au hasard, sporadique	Zufallsverteilt	Sporadico	Esporadico
Reactivity	Réactivité	Reaktivität	Reattività	Reactividad
Rhythm	Rythme	Rhythmus	Ritmo	Ritmo
Sharp and slow wave complex	*a*	Komplex aus einer steilen	Complesso onda puntuta-onda	*a*

Equivalent Terms

English	French	German	Italian	Spanish
		(scharfen) und einer langs- amen Welle	lenta	
Sharp wave	a	Steile (scharfe) Welle	Onda puntuta	Onda aguda
Sigma rhythm	Rythme sigma	Sigma-Rhythmus	Ritmo sigma	Ritmo sigma
Sigma spindle	Fuseau sigma	Sigma-Spindel	Fuso sigma	Huso sigma
Slow wave	Onde lente	Langsame Welle	Onda lenta	Onda lenta
Spike	Pointe	Spitze	Punta	Punta
Spike and wave complex	Complexe pointe onde	Spike-Wave- Komplex (S/W- Komplex)	Complesso punta-onda	Complejo punta-onda
Polyspike and wave complex	Complexe poly- pointe onde	Poly-Spike- Wave-Komplex	Complesso polipunta- onda	Complejo polipunta- onda
Spike and wave rhythm	Complexes pointe onde rhythmiques	Spike-Wave- Rhythmus (S/W- Rhythmus)	Ritmo punta- onda	Ritmo punta- onda
Theta activity	Activité thêta	Theta-Tätigkeit	Attività teta	Actividad theta
Theta rhythm	Rythme thêta	Theta-Rhythmus	Ritmo teta	Ritmo theta
Theta wave	Onde thêta	Theta-Welle	Onda teta	Onda theta
Topography	Topographie	Örtliche Verteilung	Topografia	Topografia (Dis- tribucion espacial)
Transient	Élément graphique	Einzelne über- höhte Welle	Transitorio	Fugaz
Unilateral	Unilatéral	Halbseitig	Unilaterale	Unilateral
Vertex sharp wave	Pointe vertex	Vertex-Welle	Onda puntuta al vertice	Onda aguda en vertex
Wave	Onde	Welle	Onda	Onda

aUnder discussion.

Sources of Current Information on Electronic Equipment

The electronics industry changes rapidly, and electroencephalographers must keep abreast of new developments and products. The best way to do this is to subscribe to the following periodicals, most of which are available at no cost.

General Electronic Products

"Electronic Products." United Tech. Publ., Garden City, New York.
"EEM, Electronic Engineers Master Catalog." United Tech. Publ., Garden City, New York.
"Allied Industrial Electronics Catalog." Allied Electronics, Chicago, Illinois.
"Lafayette Radio Electronics Catalog." Lafayette Radio Electronics, Syosset, Long Island, New York.

Bio-Medical Electronic Products

"Medical Instrument Dictionary and Buyers' Guide." Rimbach Publ., Pittsburgh, Pennsylvania.
"Guide to Scientific Instruments." Am. Assoc. Advan. Sci., Washington, D.C.
"Medical Electronics News." Rimbach Publ., Pittsburgh, Pennsylvania.

APPENDIX C

Recommended General Reference Books

Barnes, T. C. (1968). "Synopsis of Electroencephalography." Stechert-Hafner, New York.
Brazier, M. A. B. (1968). "The Electrical Activity of the Nervous System." Williams & Wilkins, Baltimore, Maryland.
Bureš, J., Petráň, M., and Zachar, J., eds. (1967). "Electrophysiological Methods in Biological Research," 3rd rev. ed. Academic Press, New York.
Dewhurst, D. J. (1966). "Physical Instrumentation in Medicine and Biology." Permagon Press, Oxford.
Geddes, L. A., and Baker, L. E. (1968). "Principles of Applied Biomedical Instrumentation," Wiley, New York.
Gibbs, F. A., and Gibbs, E. L. (1965). "Medical Electroencephalography." Addison-Wesley, Reading, Massachusetts.
Hill, J. D. N., and Parr, G., eds. (1963). "Electroencephalography." Macmillan, New York.
Kay, R. H. (1964). "Experimental Biology: Measurement and Analysis." Reinhold, New York.
Kiloh, L. G., and Osselton, J. W. (1961). "Clinical Electroencephalography." Butterworth, London and Washington, D.C.
Lenhoff, E. S. (1966). "Tools of Biology." Macmillan, New York.
Ochs, S. (1965). "Elements of Neurophysiology." Wiley, New York.
Offner, F. (1967). "Electronics for Biologists." McGraw-Hill, New York.
Rosenblith, W. A. ed. (1962). "Processing Neuroelectric Data." M.I.T. Press, Cambridge, Massachusetts.
Studer, J. J. (1963). "Electronic Circuits and Instrumentation Systems." Wiley, New York.
Suckling, E. E. (1961). "Bioelectricity." McGraw-Hill, New York.
Suprynowicz, V. A. (1966). "Introduction to Electronics for Students of Biology, Chemistry, and Medicine." Addison-Wesley, Reading, Massachusetts.
Anon. (1962). "A Dictionary of Electronic Terms." Allied Radio, Chicago, Illinois.
Anon. (1964). "Fundamentals of Electronics," Vol. 1, NAVPERS 93400-1. Bureau of Naval Personnel, U. S. Govt. Printing Office, Washington, D. C.

Author Index

Numbers in italics refer to the pages on which the complete references are listed.

A

Adey, W. R., 27, 28, *31*, 151, *161*, 180, 194, 217
Adrian, E. D., 20, *31*
Adrianov, O. S., 56, *71*
Ajmone-Marsan, C., 56, *72*, 174, *217*, 228, 229, 233, 236, *265*, *267*
Akert, K., 56, 65, *71*, *73*
Aladjemoff, L., 194, *222*
Albe-Fessard, D., 22, *31*
Alcaraz, M. V., 70, *72*
Andersen, P., 189, *217*
Anderson, B., 56, *71*
Anstey, N. A., 152, 154, 155, *161*
Arduini, A. A., 169, *219*
Arfel, G., 261, *267*
Arias, L. P., 186, 187, *217*, *219*
Arrigo, A., 207, *223*

B

Bachofer, C. S., 253, *267*
Bak, A. F., 54, *71*
Baker, L. E., 37, *72*
Baldwin, F., 28, *33*
Bard, P., 213, *222*
Barlow, J. S., 151, *161*
Barnes, T. C., *278*
Barry, T. J., 60, *71*
Barthel, C. A., 129, *161*
Batini, C., 194, *217*
Batsel, H. L., 199, *217*
Bauer, R. O., 200, 205, *218*
Baumgartner, G., 22, *32*
Baust, W., 205, *217*
Baylor, D., 229, *267*
Beck, E. C., 182, *217*
Beck, R. A., 142, 159, *161*
Becka, D., 227, 228, 230, *268*
Beller, A., 194, *222*
Bennett, A. E., 127, *162*
Bennett, M. V. L., 52, *71*
Benson, W. M., 206, *217*

Bethune, R. W. M., 200, *218*
Beyer, C., 177, 205, *217*
Bickford, R. G., 38, 49, *72*, 148, *161*
Bilanow, G., 52, *71*
Bleier, R., 56, *71*
Blunt, M. J., 28, *33*
Bolzani, L., 207, *223*
Bond, H. W., 20, 21, *31*
Bonnet, V., 203, *217*
Bonta, I. L., 45, *72*
Bonvallet, M., 198, 205, *217*
Bouvet, D., 209, *221*
Bradham, G. B., 142, *162*
Bradley, P. B., 48, *73*, 165, 175, 208, *217*
Brazier, M. A. B., 144, *161*, 200, 212, *217*, *278*
Brechner, V. L., 200, *218*
Bremer, F., 199, 203, *217*, *218*
Bridgman, C. S., 165, *220*
Brock, L. G., 12, 22, 23, *31*
Brodie, D. A., 201, *225*
Brody, B. S., 200, *218*
Brooks, D. C., 212, *218*
Bryce-Smith, R., 201, *218*
Buchwald, J. S., 21, *31*, 177, *218*
Buchwald, N. A., 204, *220*
Bull, J. A., 60, *71*
Bureš, J., 44, 52, 53, 56, *71*, 83, *98*, 101, 105, *126*, 142, 143, 144, *161*, 165, 193, 213, 215, *218*, *278*
Buser, P., 22, *31*, 190, *218*

C

Caceres, C. A., 96, *98*
Cadell, T. E., 253, *265*
Calma, I., 22, *33*
Candia, O., 198, *218*
Capute, A. J., 249, *267*
Carmichael, L., 165, *220*
Caspers, H., 180, *218*
Chaillet, F., 193, *223*
Chertok, I., 177, *218*
Cheshire, F. C., *161*

279

Subject Index

A

A-C, coupling of recorder amplifier, 114
Acetylcholine, 27, 208, 233
ACTH, *see* Adrenocorticotrophic hormone
Action potential, 5-7, 233-236, *see also* Multiple unit potentials
Activated EEG, *see* Desynchronization of EEG
Active transport, 2
Adrenal cortex hormones, 204
Adrenal gland, 204
Adrenocorticotrophic hormone, 204
Afterdischarge, 185, 200, 232-233, *see also* Seizures
Afterpotentials, 234
Alertness, 180, *see also* Ascending reticular arousal system
Alert wakefulness, 165-180
Alpha rhythm, 28, 90, *see also* Artifact, ocular
Amphetamine, 205, 207-208
Amphibians, 29, *see also* Frogs
Amplifiers, 103-108, 140
Amplitude, EEG characteristics of, 133-137, 143
Amplitude analysis, *see* Data analyses
Amplitude modulation, 16, 19
Amygdala, 28, 169, 172, 184, 186-187, 204
Analysis of EEG, 127-161
Anesthesia, 203, 206, 209-217, 234
  abolition of action potentials, 23
  artifact reduction, 87
  burst suppression during, 212, 216
  carbon dioxide, 201
  danger of, 240-242
  glucose effect on, 204
  local, 238
  seizure activation, 229-230, 240-241
  spindles during, 232
  use in veterinary electroencephalography, 239-240
Animals, *see* individual species

Anoxia, 199, 203, 260
Antidepressants, 207
Apical dendrites, 13, *see also* Cortex, structure of
Area postrema, and sleep, 194
Arousal, *see* Alert wakefulness, Ascending reticular arousal system
Arousal response, 167-169, 182, 185-187, 193
  blockage by tranquilizers, 207
  conditioned, 180-184
Arousal stimuli, 209
Artifact, 75-99
  ballistocardiographic, 90
  connector motion, 77, 78, 94
  electrocardiographic, 87, 88
  electrode, 35, 38
  electrode resistance effects of, 76, 78, 82
  electrostatic, EEG filters, 116
  eye movement, 90, 93, 94
  frequency band effects, 76
  general body movements, 93-98
  instrument noise as cause, 79, 121
  motion, 77, 86-98, 183-185, 238
  effect of time constants, 116-117
  muscle potentials, 87-89, 96, 97, 238
  ocular, 93-94
  physiologic, 86-98
  reduction of by use of anesthesia, 87, 242
  reference recording effects, 128-129
  respiration, 90-91
  skin potentials, 86
  ultraslow potentials, 94-95
Ascending reticular arousal system, 167, 174, 177, 186-190, 195, 205, 215, *see also* Arousal, Alert wakefulness
Asphyxia, 23
Atropine, 27, 174-175, 208
Augmenting response, 189, *see also* Recruiting response
Autocorrelation, *see also* Data analyses of EEG during anesthesia, 212
Axon, 1, 2, 4-5, 11
Axon hillock, 7

286